HEART AND BLOOD
CIRCULATORY PROBLEMS

Isabel Waugh.

1990

HEART AND BLOOD CIRCULATORY PROBLEMS

JAN DE VRIES

From the BY APPOINTMENT ONLY series

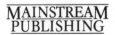

First published in 1990 by
MAINSTREAM PUBLISHING CO. (EDINBURGH) LTD
7 Albany Street
Edinburgh EH1 3UG

British Library Cataloguing in Publication Data
De Vries, Jan
  Heart and blood circulatory problems.
  1. Man. Heart. Diseases. Prevention
  I. Title   II. Series
  616.1205

  ISBN 1-85158-264-9

Typeset in 11/13 Palatino
Reproduced from disc by Polyprint, 48 Pleasance, Edinburgh, EH8 9TJ

Printed and bound in Great Britain by Billings & Sons, Worcester

Contents

Books available from the same author in the
By Appointment Only series:

Stress and Nervous Disorders (sixth impression)

Multiple Sclerosis (second impression)

Traditional Home and Herbal Remedies (third impression)

Arthritis, Rheumatism and Psoriasis (fourth impression)

Do Miracles Exist?

Neck and Back Problems (fifth impression)

Migraine and Epilepsy (second impression)

Cancer and Leukaemia (second impression)

Viruses, Allergies and the Immune System (third impression)

Realistic Weight Control

Who's Next?

Books available from the same author in the
Nature's Gift Series:

Body Energy

Foreword

A FEW YEARS ago, whilst still a medical student, I attended a somewhat unusual lecture given by a pathologist. This lecturer started off rather nervously and explained that he was going to put forward a theory which was not accepted by the orthodoxy, but felt that we would be very wise to think a little about what he was going to say. He then went on to explain how he felt that stress could produce a whole host of pathological conditions in the body, including cancer. This was thus my introduction to the many concepts of disease and illness known to us which challenge conventional and orthodox theories.

Not long afterwards, I met Jan de Vries and a vast array of different methods of diagnosis and treatment, often ignored by conventional medical training and practice, was opened up to me. These various disciplines, commonly placed under the umbrella term "alternative medicine", have fascinated me ever since and have made me examine the way medicine is organised and practised in the community and the hospitals around us.

The fact that this particular lecturer was allowed to give such a lecture to young and impressionable medical students is a sign of the change taking place in the thinking of the medical profession. This, of course, is far from universal and so very often we still encounter hostile comments from those who are less open-minded. Many patients still feel reluctant to tell their general practitioners that they are using herbal or homoeopathic remedies. I keep reminding my friends in the medical profession that many years ago herbal medicine was the *only* form of medicine available, and not the *alternative* it is seen as today.

Many readers of this book will either themselves be suffering from a heart disorder or will know of someone who is. For those affected by such problems, one of the most commonly used pharmaceutical preparations is digoxin. It is interesting to note that one of the first plants used to help those with heart problems was the foxglove, introduced by Withering in 1785 following a conversation he had with a woman who was well known for her expertise in "folk medicine". The main active component of the foxglove was later named digoxin, and it is now one of the most useful of pharmaceutical drugs used by doctors for heart problems.

In this book, Jan de Vries has covered in great detail the many aspects of heart and circulatory disorders as viewed from one side of what may be called complementary medicine. The other aspect, so very useful in the appropriate circumstance, is the side seen by cardiology departments all over the country, and many readers will be familiar with coronary care units, ECG tests, exercise tests, heart scans etc. Operations to bypass blocked arteries can be important and there is a place for this form of treatment with the right patient, but not every patient will be needing or even wanting one. There are many heart conditions where more natural and safer methods are useful and effective, but on the other hand, arguably, one of the safest places to be after a heart attack has occurred is the hospital.

There are many points of agreement between the two sides concerning the prevention, management and treatment of heart conditions that cannot be stressed enough. Diet, lifestyle, stress, smoking, etc. are extremely important and merit careful consideration. More recent research has shown that the use of fish oils can be of great benefit to those with heart complaints, something which has been believed by those practising natural medicine for a long time, based on simple observation and intuition. No doubt, much more common ground in this and other areas of medicine will be rediscovered in time.

All through the years during which I have known Jan, he has always preached that what are known as orthodox and alternative medicine must eventually meet. For the past twenty years he has worked towards the goal of achieving methods which can be complementary. Many significant steps have been made recently, and this cannot fail to be heartening for someone whose contribution to this field cannot be underestimated.

Dr Jen Tan, MB BS

1

Heart and Blood Circulation

EVERY NOW AND THEN we are sharply reminded of the fact that life ends very quickly once the heart has stopped beating. This was brought home to me and my companions a little while ago, when travelling on a Channel ferry. At a nearby table in the restaurant I noticed a gentleman who was tucking into his food with great gusto. The fact that an excellent choice of dinner or a cold self-service buffet was included in the fare may have had some bearing on the fact that this gentleman had decided to really tuck in, but looking at his girth I deduced that doing so was not unusual for him.

It must have been a sixth sense that had alerted me, because all of a sudden I saw his complexion change and he toppled over to end up lying motionless on the floor. I rushed over and helped in the effort to revive him, but to no avail. Unfortunately, this gentleman had suffered a massive heart attack and the end had been very quick.

When, eventually, the commotion had died down many passengers returned to their tables. Their meals, which had by now grown cold, were quickly whisked away and they once again made their way to the counter to choose from the wide selection of foods available before settling down to continue their meals. I sat there and studied some of them returning with heaped plates and watched them putting away enormous amounts of food, all the time talking excitedly about the unfortunate event they had witnessed only a little earlier.

I was astonished that they seemed to be quite unaware of the fact that they were effectively inflicting on themselves similar dietary mismanagement to that exhibited by the unfortunate gentleman just before he expired. I found myself wondering whether they could really be so ignorant of general dietary guidelines, or whether they were merely in a holiday mood and had temporarily decided to throw all caution to the wind.

Such an abundance or even a haphazard selection of food can easily contribute to a hardening of the arteries or to general obesity. When the first of these happens extra demands are then placed on the heart, which is required to pump the blood through restricted or less flexible arteries and veins. Obesity on its own requires more effort from the heart than would otherwise be necessary.

Do any of us ever stop to appreciate the continual task the heart mostly so faithfully performs? Do we really show this organ enough of the respect it so richly deserves? The unfortunate gentleman on the ferry may have experienced several warnings that something was wrong. He had possibly ignored those signs, but it is more likely that he was well aware that something was not quite right. If he had sought advice he might still have been there enjoying the holiday atmosphere along with his fellow passengers. Any counsellor would have pointed out to him that he was putting undue pressure on his heart by continuing to over-indulge his appetite in view of the excess weight he was already carrying.,

There is indeed much truth in the saying that we could easily eat and drink ourselves into an early grave.

The body can be regarded as a unique piece of equipment: if the maintenance and service guidelines are not adhered to, that is, a reasonable intake of food and drink and the taking of regular and sensible exercise, this equipment will not function at its optimum.

A word much bandied about nowadays is "cholesterol". It has become such a fashionable word that it appears more and more frequently on the labels of jars and bottles, especially in the case of dairy produce. Excess cholesterol often contributes to arteriosclerosis and as such endangers our health.

Only recently I returned from a most interesting visit to India, where, once again, I had seen for myself the effects of food shortages or the lack of nutritional variety. In the relatively affluent western world we have an abundance of food, a fact we so often involuntarily abuse; moreover, by doing so we endanger our health. While in the Far East and other Third World countries under-nourishment constitutes a serious health threat, we in the West could well be accused of risking our health by over-eating. The strain we place on our hearts by our modern lifestyles can be just as fatal as if we were subjected to under-nourishment. Many facets of our health are affected by gluttony, but for now I intend to concentrate on its effects on the heart.

The heart is only a small organ — barely larger than a fist — but for twenty-four hours a day, day in and day out, it ceaselessly performs a valiant task. During an average lifetime the heart pumps 500 million pints of blood through the body. Taking into account that the average body contains 8–10 pints of blood, the continual circulation of the blood through the body means that the heart pumps as much as 14,000 pints of blood daily. The lungs also play a major part by renewing the oxygen in the blood before it is pumped through the body again and again. This means that the heart beats about 100,000 times a day — almost 3,000 million times during an average lifetime. The heart muscles contract spontaneously every twenty-three seconds and the task these muscles perform can be equated to lifting a weight of 70 kg to a height of 300 metres every day. The heart depends on an intricate network of arteries, veins and capillaries which, if placed end to end, would have a total length of thousands of kilometres. These figures are very impressive, all the more so as they relate to only one of our major organs.

In days gone by, the heart was often referred to as a spiritual matter, and this does not appear to be totally unjustified in the context of emotions, shocks or fears. We have all experienced sudden palpitations when, for example, we have come to realise how narrowly we had just escaped danger by reckless driving. We also feel our heart miss a beat if we are suddenly startled out of a reverie or while we were preoccupied with another matter, and when it picks up the beat again it does so with a thump. To a certain extent I must confess to agreeing with some of the mysticism ascribed to the heart. Even the Egyptians considered the heart to be "the soul of the body". No doubt the Greeks had a more sophisticated turn of phrase for a similar idea and other civilisations also identified the heart with the life power or the spirit of the individual.

William Harvey (1578–1657), the English physician, had his own beliefs regarding the heart and when he published his conclusions on the movement of the blood by the heart he made a great impression on the medical world of his time.

Today we have well and truly reached the age of transplant surgery, but many of us can still remember when we heard about the first successful heart transplant operation. Since then the medical establishment has progressed to combined heart and lung transplants to name but one advance, and much research is still continuing. Even so, let us remember the biblical quote that "from the heart come the exits of life".

The heart fulfils a physical, mental and spiritual role in life and its functions can be encouraged and animated by following a regime of healthy food and drink intake, sensible exercise and mental stimulation through relaxation and meditation.

The incidence of coronary thrombosis is already presenting enormous problems. The occurrence of heart attacks and strokes is constantly on the increase and when we read or hear the relevant statistics we are often left wondering how we can improve our chances against falling victim to such illnesses.

As a youngster during World War II I actually ate grass to avert my hunger pains when there was no food available whatsoever. I can remember, too, seeing people collapse in the street and dying because of the lack of food and even more so the lack of adequate nutrition. Yet during those days, coronary thrombosis, heart attacks, and strokes claimed relatively few victims and the proportion of deaths attributable to heart failure or arterial problems was significantly lower than it is in our period of relative affluence.

The higher standard of living we enjoy today is certainly responsible for the present trends; in particular the tremendous increase in the use of sugar is contributory to two of the major problems, namely high blood pressure and cholesterol. Both afflictions can be countered with dietary changes. However, the increase of coronary thrombosis cannot be blamed solely on high blood pressure or lack of exercise. Factors such as tension, stress, smoking and drinking also account for the accelerated incidence of such illnesses.

It is a well-established fact that smoking is harmful. We often worry about cholesterol in the arteries but we ought to be equally if not more worried about loose particles being moved through the arteries by circulating blood.

It is a fact that smoking and drinking exacerbate such problems. There is no doubt that nicotine is harmful as it constricts the coronary arteries and therefore acts like a slow poison.

A few months ago I unexpectedly lost my brother due to heart failure while he was enjoying his annual holiday. Like me, he was brought up with the knowledge that smoking and drinking were detrimental to one's health and when at all possible my mother had raised us on a healthy and varied diet. However, during the war my brother took up smoking, initially without the knowledge of my parents, and he had continued to smoke ever since. He used to be an excellent sportsman, always remained active and throughout his life he had never lost a day's work due to illness. He had a clean record with his doctor and only a few days before setting off on his fated holiday with his wife and a couple of friends, he participated in a sponsored swim.

My brother was happily driving along in his car when suddenly his friend in the passenger seat noticed that he was losing his control over the steering wheel. This friend managed to manoeuvre the car onto the hard shoulder. My brother had suffered a massive heart attack and his death was instantaneous.

I could hardly comprehend the news when I was told. So often when we hear of the death of a family member or a friend we realise that we ought to have recognised the signs because their mental or physical activity or alertness had decreased. This had not been the case with my brother. I do, however, feel that if he had paid heed to our warnings and had stopped smoking a long time ago, he might have been able to enjoy a much longer life.

It is sensible to undergo a medical check-up every now and then. After all, when our car is three years old we take it in for an MOT test. Surely, the importance of our car cannot be less than that of our health! So often we can hear little alarm bells if we are only prepared to listen – I call it a kind of body language telling us that something is out of sorts. If we train ourselves to be attentive to them, we may be able to bring things under control before any serious harm is done. However, more often than not it seems easier to ignore such signs because of the pressure we apply to ourselves in demanding jobs and our general pace of life. It may not seem convenient just at that particular moment to make a doctor's appointment. Next week will do! But the following week we forget about it until the next warning — that is if we are lucky enough to get another warning! We owe it to ourselves to pay heed to and interpret such body language that indicates that we are on the wrong track.

To help us in this there are some simple tests and I will give further attention to these in a later chapter in this book, where I will also offer some preventative advice (see page 129). One rule, however, is to sit down after having taken some exercise and enjoy a minute's rest. Then take the pulse rate over a period of thirty seconds. Double the count of the pulse and if this is higher than 130, your exercise was too strenuous. A total count of about 100 constitutes a good level of fitness. There are quite a few simple tests and they will help us to discover our level of fitness and whether we are placing ourselves at undue risk.

If is often claimed that good health is determined by a strong and healthy heart, by clean and free-flowing blood and by unobstructed and flexible blood vessels. Of course this accounts for a sensible outlook on life, but in order to sincerely respect our health without taking it for granted, we must remind ourselves of the enormous and continual task the heart performs. Without interruption, the blood is pumped through the body, transporting oxygen and nourishment to the furthest extremities, as well as directing waste products to their destination.

Even the most competent scientist would be hard pressed to exactly identify and specify the workings of our blood circulatory system. It is stated in the Bible that "the soul is in the blood" and we must never allow ourselves to become complacent and forget how important it is to keep our blood clear and free-flowing and our circulatory system in as good a working order as we can. This "river of life" can be easily disturbed by unnatural influences, for example, drug abuse, nicotine, alcohol or an inadequate dietary regime.

It is amazing to realise the distributive function of the lymphatic or white bloodstream that is responsible for the body fluids. The so-called white bloodstream distributes leukocytes — which act as a kind of police force — and the essential lymphocytes — constituting circulatory cells.

The arteries branch out into veins, which in turn branch out into capillaries, which provide blood to each and every cell in the body; together, these vessels cover an enormous distance. This system deserves our full support to keep this magnificent function in optimum working order and if we take sufficient care, we ourselves will be the beneficiaries. If, on the other hand, we allow the condition of our blood to decline, our health will undoubtedly decline too. It is the purpose of this book to direct the reader towards ways in which we can take the necessary care to maintain a good circulation and from the following chapters it will become clear how important a role our lifestyle plays in this respect.

2

Angina

IT HAD FIRST started with a little constricting pain that my patient had tried, unsuccessfully, to ignore, together with a gradual tightening of the throat. His wife's comments had been to the effect that he was always complaining and most likely the problem was all in the mind. When he became unable to shut the pain out of his mind he had decided to come and see me without his wife's knowledge. Initially, on listening to the summing up of his symptoms, I wondered whether his wife might perhaps be right. He certainly looked well enough and there seemed to be no visible signs indicating that anything was out of order. Nevertheless, on my advice he did go to see his general practitioner and the early signs he had experienced were consequently diagnosed as angina.

The early symptoms of angina could quite easily be overlooked and dismissed as a minor discomfort. If ignored, this condition could easily develop into a full-blown angina pectoris displaying not only the aforementioned symptoms but also a painful tightening in the chest caused by a restriction in the supply of blood to the heart. This again is often conveniently explained away as a muscular strain.

Some time ago I had diagnosed a middle-aged to elderly female patient as suffering from all the symptoms of angina and stressed the importance of her seeking her general practitioner's help. Afterwards, I learned that she had not taken my advice and within six months she had died from heart failure. So often I see that apparently minor discomforts are brushed aside without a second thought, while later they are found to have been the first tell-tale signs of a serious illness. It is difficult to draw the line between when one might be considered a hypochondriac and when it is wise to make further investigations. The body will always let us know if something is not quite right, but please do not become neurotic about every little sign of a minor discomfort. Learn to listen to the language of your own body because usually it is a combination of seemingly unconnected and trivial irregularities that point towards a more major disorder. Any persistent, niggling complaints could well amount to an early warning system. If this happens to you, do something about it.

Such niggles can be the onset of angina or related problems that may have been developing over a period of time, but it is also possible that such a condition can hit us suddenly. Whichever way it strikes us it is a warning that there is something out of order with the heart and that the heart and/or the coronary arteries that carry the blood to the heart muscles might be exhausted, depleted or even suffering from a breakdown. Heart disease is a major problem in the United Kingdom and especially so in certain parts of Scotland, where an unusually high incidence of heart problems has been found to occur. This is possibly due to dietary ignorance or an unwillingness to decrease the intake of fats, sugar and related food products which do not benefit the major chamber of the heart.

Very often, more serious complaints can be averted by taking timely measures to stimulate the flow of oxygen and so improve the heart circulation. I am sure that the total of 100,000 coronary bypass operations undertaken each year in the United States could be greatly reduced if some protective measures were taken in the early stages or, better still, before any warning signs become apparent. Nor would it surprise me if 60 per cent of the cases of heart surgery for coronary vessel disease in the United Kingdom could be avoided or at least drastically reduced by paying more attention to the early signs.

Such was the case with an elderly gentleman who came to our clinic for acupuncture therapy. During his treatment he appeared somewhat agitated and the colour of his complexion deepened. When I checked his blood pressure etc. I realised his condition and together we worked out a few minor adjustments to his lifestyle. He now lives happily with these changes and his health is much improved.

There is no need to wait for the gripping severity of pain which can occur from time to time. It is in the early stages that we can most effectively prevent the situation from becoming too serious. The heart, that remarkable piece of equipment that pumps the life blood through our arteries and veins, deserves our admiration and consideration and the vessels that carry the blood to the muscle walls can well do with a bit of a rest from time to time. As I have said before, we take our car in for an MOT test and obtain a certificate of roadworthiness, and this finely tuned piece of equipment, which works continuously throughout our life, at least deserves similar consideration to that shown to our car. Basically, it all rests with common sense and, as I never tire of pointing out, there is nothing common about common sense!

The early symptoms of angina may be a slight tingling

of the lips, or a fairly persistent dull headache, or even some problems with the vision; all of these indicate a rise in the blood pressure, which causes a strain to be placed on the heart. The blood may contain tiny particles that have been formed as a result of poor dietary management and these particles can clog, narrow or obstruct the arteries. Yet again, there are ways in which such conditions can be overcome.

On one occasion I examined a middle-aged lady who appeared to be suffering from some early angina symptoms and I explained that her heart was beating some forty million times a year and that in seventy years the labour of pumping the blood through the body about 3,000,000,000 pulsations were required. Sceptically, she looked at me and asked, "What has this to do with me being overweight?" I had to tell her that, unfortunately, her heart was already protesting and that she was clearly showing early symptoms of angina. To encourage the life motor — her heart — to continue doing its task, it would be essential to reduce her weight. I enquired whether she suffered from indigestion and whether wind caused her pain around the chest area and hesitantly she agreed that this was the case.

So very often I notice that symptoms such as indigestion, wind and flatulence, all of which are small alarm signals in their own way, are conveniently misinterpreted or ignored. This poor lady was puffing and panting at the thought of having to go on a diet. When I asked her if she had any constipation problems she proudly denied this, adding that she passed a motion every second or third day. She was most indignant when I told her that one is undeniably constipated if one does not have a daily bowel movement. In my lectures I often stress the point that what is imported into the body over a period of twenty-four hours also ought to be exported within a similar time span.

On another occasion I was consulted by a lady who

asked me if I would please give her osteopathic treatment for her neck. Before doing so I asked to take her blood pressure. As I expected this was found to be sky high: with a weight of 21 stones while she had not yet reached the age of thirty, her blood pressure reading was 220 over 140. I could only pray that I could instil some sense into her before it was too late. I also asked her about the regularity of her bowel movements and she told me that on average she had a bowel movement once a week. I lectured her on the severity of her condition and advised her of some measures she could introduce immediately, but I also stressed the need for her to make an appointment to see her general practitioner. When she came back to the clinic two weeks later a considerable improvement in her blood pressure was already apparent and she thanked me for "putting the wind up her" because she felt quite a bit happier for finally having done something about her weight instead of postponing the evil day when the problem had to be faced. I was then more than willing to give her the manipulation treatment she had requested for her neck problems.

As is so often the case, the build-up of fluid puts unnecessary strain on the heart, causing dizziness and headaches indicating that something is not as it should be. In most cases fluid retention will diminish when a sensible dietary regime is adopted.

I have already touched on some of the causes of angina and the causes of overloading the heart and I have pointed out that these problems often develop over a period of time, as the symptoms of angina rarely appear until there is an artery closure of around 90–95 per cent. Hence my insistence upon a sensible approach to diet and exercise and the reduction of stress and other factors that could easily be contributory to producing angina complaints.

Smoking will increase the levels of noradrenalin, which is a hormone that contributes to the maintenance of the circulatory and nervous system. It is well known that nicotine is contributory to angina problems. So is alcohol and some of the drugs that, unfortunately, are becoming so popular. I always attempt to take the time to look at the personality of a patient who is suspected of having heart problems; I study their emotions and so try to decide on their temperament. Angina patients often appear to be emotional, volatile, quick to cry, occasionally somewhat aggressive and nearly always very impatient. In fact, these could be considered as the characteristics of the average angina patient, although of course hereditary factors cannot be ignored. Yet I have found that it always pays to study the characteristics of a heart patient in order to be able to best advise him or her.

Admittedly, it is not always simple to change our lifestyle, but if we consider that we have no option if we want to continue living, then doing so must surely be considered a challenge.

Again, I come back to my brother's claims that he had never missed a day's work through illness and never had reason to consult a doctor. He always seemed to be full of vigour, yet he had ignored the unquestionable tell-tale signs. These came to light after his demise and the post mortem concluded that he had suffered a massive heart attack due to a progressive angina.

Nutritional research has shown that certain vitamins, minerals and trace elements are often deficient in angina sufferers. Recently I read a paper on a study of this subject, which indicated that patients with these problems have a lower level of PLP, an active metabolic form of pyridoxine. This not only represents a risk factor such as high blood pressure — a possible cause for heart disease — but it also seems that such patients have a low level of vitamin B_6.

Then there is the question of vitamin E. A short while ago a colleague phoned me about an angina patient who had a severe tachycardia. He was considering hospitalising him but as he knew that I was well acquainted with the patient he asked me about his high intake of vitamin E. He wondered if the patient's daily intake of 1,200 IU of vitamin E might have any bearing on the occurrence of tachycardia. He was, indeed right to question this because even though vitamin E is a wonderful vitamin that can be safely used by heart and angina patients, I advise people to never exceed the level of 600 IU daily. This, taken in combination with oil of evening primrose, will bring about a definite improvement in one's condition.

There is, however, always the question of what level of vitamin intake is beneficial and when do we reach the point where we are overdoing things? A recent survey, conducted with the co-operation of more than 250 health food stores, reached the conclusion that there was no easy standard answer to this question, but that the most beneficial level varied according to the individual. The logical conclusion, therefore, must be that one ought to steer on the side of caution; however, under careful monitoring by medically trained persons a higher dosage may occasionally be taken depending on the circumstances.

An interesting paper was presented at a seminar on vitamin E held in Colorado in June 1989. Professor Anthony Diplock, Head of the Department of Biochemistry at the United Medical and Dental School of Guy's and St Thomas' Hospitals in London, presented a paper about the recent findings of two researchers, Adrianne Bendich, PhD, and Learns G. Machlin, PhD. Amongst the conclusions reached by Bendich and Machlin were the following:

—The toxicity of vitamin E is low.
—Animal studies have shown no mutagenic (changes in cellular structure), carcinogenic, or teratogenic (foetal change) effects of vitamin E.

—In double-blind human studies with large population groups, oral supplements of vitamin E resulted in few if any undesirable side-effects.

So, while 200–400 IU remains the most popular daily intake, the good news, in Professor Diplock's words, is: "Vitamin E is very safe up to a quite massive dosage."

At the same seminar a possible link between vitamin E and the prevention of heart disease was discussed by Dr Hermann Esterbauer of the University of Graz, whose experiments have helped to elucidate how low-density lipoproteins (LDLs) become converted to plaque-producing foam cells via oxidation. This is one of the early steps in the development of cardiovascular disease. Vitamin E may be one of the body's key players in preventing the atherogenic modification of LDLs.

Researchers in France tested this theory on human beings and found that vitamin E did indeed help to prevent the modification of LDLs into the oxidised o-LDLs bound for fatty streaks and plaques on artery walls.

A Swiss researcher, Dr K. Fred Gey, reported on epidemiological data from several European nations, which showed a correlation between higher blood levels of vitamin E and lower rates of heart disease.

As a protector of the fats in cell membranes (and therefore of the integrity of the cell), vitamin E plays a particularly important role in the health of the nervous system, which is very rich in fats. Vitamin E deficiency diseases are characterised by neuropathy, or disorders of the peripheral nerves, as well as the deterioration of the spinal cord.

Certain vitamin combinations are recommended for heart and angina patients and in this context I would not hesitate to suggest that a patient use the Chelation Formula from Nature's Best. This is a simple and effective combination of chelating nutrients from natural sources. Two tablets taken daily will provide an ideal supplement for city dwellers and those who work near chemical and nuclear plants.

Co-Enzyme Q10 (Co–Q10) falls in the same category. It gets to the heart of our energy production system, since this enzyme is found in the mitochondria of all living cells. The mitochondria are the energy generators of cells. The highest proportion of mitochondria are found in those cells that do the most work. Not surprisingly, these occur in the liver, in muscle tissue and in the heart. Co–Q10 was discovered by the Nature's Best consultant Dr Len Mervyn. New technology has recently made it possible to provide meaningful amounts of Co–Q10 in supplement form, and researchers are still uncovering the full potential of what leading scientists call the "biochemical spark" that releases energy.

Co–Q10 is found in certain foods, but has proved difficult to extract from them. It is synthesised in the body and our ability to either absorb or produce it deteriorates as we age. Nutritional deficiencies and genetic or acquired defects can also interfere with the Co–Q10 metabolic pathway — a pathway that results in physical energy.

Because Co–Q10 enables the body to use oxygen effectively and is so important for the hardest-working organs and tissues of the body, athletes are among those who may choose it as a supplement. In Japan and the United States, where clinical research into Co–Q10 is well advanced, it has been used in efforts to support energy production in the heart muscle.

Many of us take it for granted that heart problems will only strike the older generation, but we must realise that this is not necessarily so. I remember a lady who had not yet reached thirty when she already displayed all the symptoms of angina pectoris. We checked her medical history and discovered that, due to certain circumstances, her diet had gone totally haywire and the balance had totally disappeared. Indeed, this factor proved to be one of the main reasons for the problems she had recently been experiencing. Fortunately, this lady recognised the seriousness of the situation and together we made some adjustments to her diet and with the help of some essential fatty acids combined with vitamin E and a number of homoeopathic remedies we managed to reverse her condition and avert the danger of impending heart disease.

It is necessary to consider the characteristics of angina and align these with the various homoeopathic remedies available and then study the kind of person and the symptoms. If heart cramps are the problem because of oxygen starvation, the advice will often be to take the homoeopathic potency *Tabacum* 6x for acute and serious cases, while for chronic conditions *Tabacum* 12x will be prescribed. For conditions including heart cramps this remedy has been found to be most useful. The same remedy may also be used quite safely and effectively in cases of constriction of the coronary arteries. In cases of imminent collapse, indicated by cold sweat on the forehead and pain in the legs, *Veratrum album* 6x is most helpful and Arnica 30x will be beneficial when the heart also needs some strengthening. If the patient is high in colour or blushes, then we can use Naya 12x.

Then there are the Dr Vogel remedies Crataegisan and *Viscum album*. Crataegisan is a fresh herb preparation for nervous heart problems, a senile heart, heart stress, myocardial weakness following injections, palpitations and feelings of anxiety. The main ingredient of this remedy is *Crataegus oxyacantha* or the hawthorn berry.

Should constipation be a problem then we might use the Vogel remedy Linoforce. This is a mild natural laxative that helps give temporary relief from occasional constipation and increases the frequency of bowel movements. It helps to regulate the intestinal activity and acts as a stool softener. This is a herbal remedy with flaxseed and senna leaves as its main components.

For a really old-fashioned but effective remedy for constipation take my grandmother's advice: eat some grapes every day, but do not discard the pips because they must be chewed. So often I see people taking out the pips, but these are most effective when chewed. Do not let it bother you that this advice appears too simple to be true because it really is most effective.

In his excellent book *The Nature Doctor* Dr Alfred Vogel describes an old country remedy for cramps and especially for angina and similar conditions this has proved to be very effective. From this book I quote:

> Generally speaking, bad heart cramps are relieved only by strong medicines, usually Amylnitrite or Trinitrini. There is, however, an old exceedingly simple remedy which is quite easy to come by. It relieves cramp pains and leaves no aftermath or complications. It is good for a cramp in asthma cases too. This is an old peasant remedy which has been in use for centuries but now, alas, it is almost forgotten.
>
> Take fermented cider, the older the better, heat it until it reaches boiling point and quickly remove it from the fire. Soak some towels in hot cider and place them as hot as they can be borne on both arms, covering each arm completely. The heat plus the fruit acids of the hot cider will decongest the heart circulation, soothe the blood vessels and the nervous system and relieve the cramps. This simple method can be augmented by putting a hot linseed, hay flower or lemon balm compress on the heart.
>
> Cramp-like conditions brought about by angina pectoris or other similar causes follow the course of the sympathetic nerve. Very often they begin in the pit of the stomach near the sternum and move up the neck leaving a feeling almost amounting to strangulation. Such distressing conditions will be relieved in a remarkable way if the suggestions made above are followed.

Although the above remedies and methods will prove helpful, it is nevertheless important that the angina patient checks on the stress and emotional factors affecting his or her life. The word "stress" currently appears to be in vogue. Especially for the angina sufferer, stress can certainly induce many unnecessary problems. It may be caused by unhappiness, marital problems, unemployment or anything that causes excessive worry. Sometimes we cannot even identify the exact cause. Stress-related problems increase the strain on the heart to such an extent that in some cases I have seen this to be fatal.

A sound remedy for reducing stress is found in *Avena sativa* or Avenaforce. This is a fresh herb preparation for strengthening the nerves and relieving insomnia and irritability. It relaxes and promotes falling asleep and its main ingredient is fresh oat seed. This remedy invariably helps to reduce stress and can always be used safely without fear of adverse side-effects.

Simple relaxation exercises are another useful means of reducing stress. There are few better in this respect than the Hara breathing method. I have already described this method in my book on *Stress and Nervous Disorders*, but for those of you who are not familiar with this I will do so again below.

Years ago, when I was working in a particular hospital, I could not fail to notice that one young doctor there was able to perform more operations than any of her colleagues and she still looked relaxed at the end of the day. I asked her what her secret was and she replied that all she did was try to breathe correctly in order to have an energy supply to draw on whenever the need arose. She explained that although her method was simple, it still required a fair amount of practice.

Where does a young baby breathe from? If you look, you will find that there is little movement of the chest and there is a rhythmic rise and fall slightly below the navel. As the child grows older and forms its own personality, this breathing pattern will change, usually rising from the navel upwards. In adults, tense people tend to breathe high up in the chest and the same can be said for those suffering from asthma.

The young doctor then told me that her breathing technique was based on "Hara" and to this day I am grateful that I managed to receive some instruction into this method of correct breathing. The technique involves too many exercises for me to include them all here, but I will tell you about one specific exercise that I myself practise almost daily.

At about four o'clock, the time of day I was born, I sometimes begin to feel a little tired. This, by the way, is a feeling experienced by many people when the time of their birth approaches. I lie down on the floor when I feel tired and tell myself to relax completely. With my eyes closed, I concentrate on relaxing every part of my body, from top to toe. Eventually, I feel as if I am sinking deeper and deeper into the floor. Then I place my left hand about half an inch beneath my navel and put the other hand on it. At that point a magnetic ring on the vital centre of man — Hara — is formed. The Chinese have an old saying that the navel is the gate to all happiness and certainly, by doing this, one feels very relaxed. Next I breathe in slowly through the nose, filling my stomach with air and keeping the rib cage still. This sounds easier than it is and actually takes a little time and concentration to master properly. Once the stomach is filled with air, I round my lips and slowly breathe out, pulling the stomach flat.

This exercise can be done as often as desired. Normally, the sensation after finishing this exercise is either one of complete relaxation and the desire for a nice sleep, or of refreshment and the desire to return to work. I must stress that it should be performed naturally, as a baby might do it. When you first try this exercise do not give up too soon if you do not feel any immediate effect, because it takes some time to get into the swing of it. It will be worth your while to persevere because it is a marvellous relaxation exercise.

There are, of course, other ways to reduce stress, such as yoga, autogenic training or meditation, but whichever method suits you best or appeals most, let it be a relaxation exercise. Should none of these methods be sufficiently effective then you will need to programme yourself differently and determinedly set out to ensure that enough time is allocated for rest, relaxation and sleep. Consciously try and take life easier.

Sound sleep is clearly of great benefit in reducing stress and is also essential to our well-being. We all go through spells when our sleeping pattern appears to be disrupted, but we should always take care not to become dependent on sleeping tablets or other drugs. Here again the Hara breathing method can be useful. In addition, some natural remedies such as Dormeasan from Dr Vogel will ensure a good rest. Dormeasan is a fresh herb preparation for mild sleeping disorders and stress. It has a calming effect and is also used to counter over-excitement, restlessness, nervous exhaustion as well as mental over-exertion. It is prepared from the following ingredients:

Melissa off.	— balm
Avena sativa	— oats
Passiflora incarnata	— Passion flower
Humulus lupulus	— hops
Valeriana off.	— valeria
Lupulinum	— hop grains

And then there is the oxygen factor. Try to develop the habit of regularly taking a brief walk. There is no need to go on long hikes, but make sure it is a walk in the fresh air and inhale deeply to fill the lungs with the oxygen your body needs so badly.

Angina patients often complain of pain in the neck, shoulders and/or upper arms. Here some gentle massage may well be received gratefully, but if that opportunity does not exist I can wholeheartedly recommend some of Dr Bach's flower remedies. Reflexology or aromatherapy can also be useful for such problems. In my book *Body Energy* I have described several methods that can be very useful to an angina patient and some of these could well be adapted to relieve such pains and ease any strains.

Not only is diet important to an angina patient but digestion is too. I have already made the point that we should ensure that we do not become constipated, but many people may not be aware of the fact that indigestion expresses itself in our posture and that many posture defects are the result of poor digestion. Most healthy people enjoy a well-functioning digestive system. As soon as problems arise in this field a person's general well-being will be affected and the posture will often serve as an indication of that person's general health. A brief description of each of the various postures and its possible causes is given below:

Normal posture
The position and volume of the stomach and bowels are normal, and therefore the person sits or stands straight. When relaxed, the chest will be somewhat barrel-shaped. Unless the contents of the stomach are too heavy, the sternum and the pubic bone should be aligned.

Salute posture
Due to a heavy stomach and abdomen, the upper section of the spine is straight. The chest is expanded, the midriff high and the pelvis will be tilted forward.

Take-off posture
This is caused by chronically weakened bowels and enlarged stomach contents requiring an increased stomach area. The upper spine is stretched and shows a tendency to lean forward.

Duck posture

Because of fairly severe digestive problems, a larger stomach area is required, causing a forward tilt of the pelvis (or a protrusion of the backside), and a broadening and lifting of the chest. (Watch out, too, for a shortening of the neck.)

Sagging posture

People with weak muscles and an irregular bowel movement pattern, necessitating an enlarged area for the stomach contents, often display a rounded upper spine and dropped stomach.

Sower posture

Severe chronic weakening of the bowels and swelling caused by a build up of faeces results in a low-slung stomach (comparable to the sower who carries a bag of seeds in front of him). Due to the weight of the sagging stomach, the upper body will be inclined to compensate and will lean backwards.

Drummer posture

This posture can be attributed to a considerable increase in the bowel contents due to irregular bowel movements and flatulence. The digestive system is severely handicapped. The considerable broadening and a general lifting of the chest appears to make the neck sink between the shoulders. This posture is only possible when there is a convex spinal curvature and a tilting forward of the pelvis.

The points listed below can be used as a checklist to help determine whether the digestive system is functioning normally.

—No eructions or stomach acid?

—No haemorrhoids, blockage or gall problems?
—No distended stomach because of flatulence?
—No sensitive appendix (due to inert digestion)?
—No rheumatism (a sign of the presence and build up of
  digestive poisons in the tissue)?
—No pains in the abdomen caused by a forward tilt of the
  pelvis?

Another point to check is whether there is a regular daily bowel movement. This should be neither too stodgy nor thin, nor should it smell too strongly, and it should be passed without besmirching the anus.

The postures described on pages 33-34 may well be helpful in discovering where particular problems stem from. Once this is known, then something can be done about it. Therefore I will follow the above advice with a proposed diet. When people hear the word "diet" they mostly associate it with an attempt at weight reduction. If, however, you have recognised yourself in the description of any of the postures above, or if you already know that your digestive system leaves something to be desired, the following diet may be helpful. In other words, it is a health-promoting diet rather than a weight-reducing diet, but it cannot fail to improve your feeling of well-being.

Breakfast
Muesli prepared by mixing together or liquidising the following ingredients:
—1 tablespoon oats (whole oats from a health food store
— or use flakes of wheat, rye, barley, etc.) soaked overnight in water
—1 grated apple
—1 other portion of fruit, e.g. pear, grapes, apricots (if
  dried soaked overnight in water)
—2 tablespoons natural yoghurt
—1 tablespoon quark or "fromage frais"

—honey to taste
—3 almonds, 3 hazelnuts, 10 pumpkin seeds, 10 sunflower seeds

Lunch

Use three different raw vegetables per meal chosen from within groups 1, 2 or 3:

Group 1: Carrot, red beetroot, radish, garlic, onion, celeriac, black radish, swede

Group 2: Cucumber, cauliflower, broccoli, celery, leek, fennel, pepper, tomatoes

Group 3: Lettuce, white cabbage, red cabbage, spinach, watercress, chicory, endive, iceberg lettuce

Dressing for raw vegetables:
—2-3 tablespoons yoghurt
—1 tablespoon Molkosan
—onion and/or garlic
—herbs

To accompany the raw vegetables choose one of the following:
—jacket potato
—brown rice
—two slices of crispbread
—one slice of pumpernickel or ryebread

Dinner

Muesli — see breakfast recipe
Vegetable soup made from fresh vegetables
Salad
Potatoes (small amount)

Beverages

Herbal tea or Bambu coffee
Drink one or two cups of fresh carrot juice daily

Do not eat
Chocolate, cheese (you can have cottage cheese), eggs, cream, cow's milk (have soya milk instead), butter, processed foods, white flour, refined sugar (or products made with them), pork (in any form), citrus fruits, coffee, red wine, excess alcohol, vinegar, tea, smoked or pickled foods, animal fats, spices

General advice
Do not eat after 8.00 p.m.
If hungry between meals or after 8.00 p.m. have an apple or some other fruit
Make sure you chew your food well
Smoking is prohibited

Every single patient will express the desire to get back to normal, in other words to return to the state of health they used to enjoy. Fortunately, I have seen many of them achieve a considerable improvement once they have appreciated their condition and have taken the effort to do something about it before it is too late. I understand that it can be frustrating when you are told to take things easier for the time being, but, with care, you can be instrumental in improving your general condition and so able to enjoy good health once more. It often requires only minor adjustments and your body will gratefully repay you for the encouragement you have given it.

3

Heart Attacks

LET US NOW look into the question I so often hear: "What really is a heart attack?" The simplest reply to this question is that an obstruction in the flow of blood to one or more of the coronary arteries and degeneration in the muscle fibres of those muscles will cause atrophy. When the muscles that are deprived of oxygen cease to function correctly a heart attack may well occur; its severity will depend on how large an area of the heart muscle is affected.

It is, of course, not easy to determine the severity of such a heart attack. Some heart attacks can be fairly minor and are therefore barely noticed. The right and left coronary arteries can be affected individually to a greater or lesser extent. As the coronary arteries branch out into smaller vessels to supply blood to the heart muscles, a blockage of a tiny vessel can mean that only a small part of the heart may be deprived of blood, whereas a blockage in a major vein or artery will usually affect a much larger part of the heart muscle. When the blood cannot flow unhindered to supply the heart and to remove waste, then chemicals can build up and the heart can come under severe pressure.

Statistics show that in 1982 heart attacks accounted for 31 per cent of all male deaths in Britain. Deaths due to cancer accounted for 24 per cent and strokes were responsible for 9 per cent. The mortality rate for males between the ages of thirty-five and sixty appeared to be 30–40 per cent higher in Scotland than in England, which makes me wonder if the high percentage of heart attacks in Scotland may be due to diet. Moreover, I am a firm believer that it is also related to the use of alcohol and nicotine.

Among females the percentages are somewhat different. Deaths due to heart disease accounted for 23 per cent of the total, while strokes accounted for 15 per cent. However, clogged-up arteries were responsible for 38 per cent of the female mortality and it is estimated that in Britain heart disease claims a total of 200,000 deaths each year. I consider dietary habits as the major cause for concern underlying these grave statistics. It does not require great mathematical expertise to reach this conclusion because dietary management has clearly undergone great changes.

During my travels I have noticed that in the Far East heart attacks are much less common than in the West, and I have found it interesting to study the difference in the dietary habits of these countries I have visited there. They have a very much lower intake of sugar and obtain much of their nourishment from vast amounts of natural unpolished rice. In some of the countries where seaweed is regularly featured on the menu, I have also found it most encouraging to see that the incidence of heart failure is much lower than in the West.

It is also largely true that people who perform hard physical work and those who are not overweight are much less likely to develop heart disease. I remember

Dr Alfred Vogel once relating to me a discussion he had had with some elderly physicians. They had told him that heart disease among their patients was largely unknown, despite the fact that the physicians all had rural practices and the majority of their patients performed manual labour. This would seem to confirm that mental stress is much more likely to trigger off a heart attack than, for example, a hard day's physical work in the garden. We should not forget the importance of oxygen either. I agree that it often seems much more convenient to take the car rather than using our legs for the purpose they were designed for. However, due to lack of physical exercise the blood circulatory system will become less efficient and this could contribute to a deterioration of the vascular system, as well as the heart. A heart attack may eventually be the result of such negligence. In some cases a minor heart attack is not always such a bad thing as it could well serve as a serious warning that it may soon be too late to mend our ways and change our habits.

People who fall between the ages of forty-five and sixty-five in particular would do well to realise that if they take insufficient physical exercise and are employed in a stressful occupation, heart seizures, heart cramps or a heart attack will be more likely to occur. Those people would be wise to look at possible ways of adapting their lifestyles so as to reduce the risk of suffering a heart attack.

Any signs or symptoms experienced which point in this particular direction indicate a need to have such problems investigated, so as to ensure that the vascular system is in reasonably good order and that no other influences are serving to increase the risk of a heart attack. Problems such as hyperventilation or other symptoms that might be attributed to heart disease in general must be checked, if for no other reason than to allow the individual to banish such negative fears from the mind.

The other day a patient told me that for the last three years she had imagined more or less daily that she had fallen prey to a heart attack. In her case I could easily reassure her that if that had been the case she would not be sitting opposite me talking to me about it. If you are experiencing such fears, always have them investigated to establish whether there is any basis for them and to put your mind at rest. Fear can be a formidable enemy and, unfortunately, can even lead to the birth of the problem that was so much feared in the first place. Always attempt to maintain a positive outlook and, if it makes you feel better, seek professional advice. Try not to worry about what happened yesterday, because most fears are rooted in the past anyway. Nor is it wise to worry about what may lie ahead of us because those fears may never come to pass.

Another problem I often encounter is the anxiety that is so often experienced by the real heart patient. Anxiety can be the result of excessive stress and tension, but it is equally true that it can be induced by negative thoughts. Patients who suffer from anxiety must be treated with consideration, patience and understanding and every effort should be made to discover the cause for this anxiety. If we live life under a cloud because we suspect that the first heart attack was a warning and therefore the next one is going to be the big one, our fears are more likely to bring about what we dread most. Again, my advice would be to adopt a positive attitude and try to overcome such fears and anxieties and, wherever possible, to do something constructive in order to avert such dangers.

Modern society has much to answer for and there is little doubt about the root cause of our diminished resistance to some of the attacks being made on our health. Our society has treated the sources of the basic energies of life with a total disregard, these energies being food, water and air. Through pollution the nature of these basic energies has changed; instead of being conducive to health they are now sometimes considered as endangering our health. Most of you will know that air is made up of oxygen (20 per cent) and nitrogen (78 per cent) together with a few minor traces of other gases. The circulatory system is highly dependent on oxygen and a regular and unhindered supply of oxygen is most important if we are to protect ourselves against heart attacks. Deprivation of oxygen can cause circulatory failure, while a severe shortage of oxygen will cause a heart attack and perhaps even death. Inhaling oxygen will always effect an improvement and to this extent exercises, meditation or relaxation could well prove helpful.

Patients who have previously suffered a heart attack derive tremendous benefits from the use of certain remedies that aid the transport of oxygen. I can especially recommend remedies containing vitamin E because it produces collagen, a structural protein that consolidates the cells and so helps the heart muscle and other connective tissues to maintain their functions. Bioflavonoids aid the absorption of vitamin C and help to maintain a healthy bloodstream and blood vessels, and like vitamin C itself, have anti-oxidant capabilities.

Dr Christian Barnard, who performed the world's first heart transplant operation, did not believe that jogging or physical exercise provided any benefit to people. He also advised his patients to follow a diet that was quite high in cholesterol. His most successful patient lived for a period of nineteen months after the transplant operation, but I am quite sure that if this patient had followed a diet that was lower in cholesterol and had taken exercise to encourage the supply of oxygen, he might well have lived considerably longer.

Another aspect of heart disease is the disruption of the rhythm by impaired muscle co-ordination. It is important that a heart patient leads a regular, harmonious and programmed life. Sufficient rest must be taken and enough time should be allowed for meals. Very often a heart attack will take place late at night or after midnight and this is not surprising when we consider that most people take their main meal during early or mid evening. Usually, the meal is too rich for that time of night and it is often accompanied by alcohol and/or the use of nicotine. This combination can induce indigestion or absorption problems which speed up the normal heart rate and create stress.

When we are under stress the nervous system is jolted and a heart attack or some fibrillation or fluttering can occur, instead of the normal pumping action of the heart. If susceptible to the latter, it is often decided to fit such a patient with a pacemaker; a minute battery is implanted to regulate the patient's heartbeat and so give him or her the chance to lead as normal a life as possible.

I have already touched on some aspects of what happens during a heart attack and what measures can be taken to reduce the risk factor. Even if a heart attack has already occurred there are still ways to minimise the risk of a repeat attack. If no heart attack has yet taken place, we would still be wise to follow this advice as prevention is better than cure. It should always be remembered that the responsibility lies with the individual and cannot be passed on to someone else.

Smoking and drinking are never beneficial to our health and these habits or addictions can be overcome with some common sense and willpower. Overcoming obesity may be somewhat more difficult and here one can seek dietary advice. One can even decide to resort to acupuncture treatment or some of the other available ways to find the encouragement that is sometimes needed. Inadequate exercise, high levels of stress and negative emotions must be carefully looked at and steps taken to remedy these. Heart attacks can be enormously debilitating and will out of necessity result in a different lifestyle, so it would be in our own best interests to look at preventative measures, while we still have the chance.

The electrical system of the heart is controlled by the sino-atrial node and the atrio-ventricular node. The blood supply is gained from the right coronary artery and if the small branches of this system become blocked, the harmonious rhythm is disturbed and rapid treatment may be called for. In such instances I have seen great results when Dr Bach's Rescue Remedy has been used — a combination of flower remedies. This also applies to Dr Vogel's Cardiaforce, a tonic that contains extracts from the following herbs:

Crataegus oxyacantha	— hawthorn berry
Avena sativa	— oats
Arnica montana	— arnica
Cactus grandiflorus	— blooming cereus
Lycopus europaeus	— bugleweed
Ilex aquifolium	— holly
Passiflora incarnata	— passion flower
Spiritus camphoratus	— camphor

Cardiaforce is a tonic for nervous heart disorders, palpitations, rapid heartbeat and sensations of constriction. It promotes circulation in the cardiovascular system and calms an over-excited or over-stimulated heart.

About a third of all people who suffer a heart attack are suspected to be suffering from angina and most of these will have experienced some kind of warning, whether or not they have interpreted the signs correctly. The pain that accompanies a heart attack is mostly of a sudden onset and is similar to angina pain. However, the pain will often be more persistent and can usually be relieved with medication. If no medication is available immediate action is essential. When the patient experiences pain in the chest together with sweating, giddiness, breathing difficulties, a sickly feeling or even vomiting, instant help is needed. In the Far East I learned about a simple method that can be applied in such instances. Cross the arms of the patient and gently, but quite firmly, rub the pulse where it can be felt on the wrist. Loosen tight clothing at the throat and across the chest and waist. Place some cold cloths on the nape of the neck or on the forehead. Keep on rubbing the pulse and this may well save the patient's life until a medically trained person can take charge.

Always remember how important it is that proper care is taken of intestinal activities; we should always try to maintain regular bowel movements and, above all, follow a sensible diet. Let me point again to the benefits of natural unpolished rice and raw fruit and vegetables. Vitamin E is helpful and may be taken in the form of wheatgerm oil. Also remember that salt intake should be kept to a minimum.

Among the range of remedies from Dr Vogel there are also two herbal remedies that I can wholeheartedly recommend: Arterioforce and *Viscum album*.

Arterioforce is specifically designed for people who suffer from hardening of the arteries and early signs of senility. It serves to ease the effects of arteriosclerosis and increases the capacity for activity. It is also suitable for the treatment of complaints such as tiredness, listlessness, loss or weakness of memory, dizziness, slightly elevated blood pressure, reduced concentration and loss of vitality.

Viscum album is a fresh herb preparation (see page 102) for arteriosclerosis, cases of extreme hypertension and neurasthenia. It particularly stimulates the cell metabolism in cases of nervous advanced age syndrome.

In later chapters of this book I will give some diets that are designed to counter specific conditions, but in this instance follows a general diet.

Breakfast
Dr Vogel's Breakfast Muesli with the juice of an orange, a grated apple, half a banana, or other fruit.

One or two pieces of rye crispbread or wholemeal bread spread with natural vegetable (sunflower or corn-oil) margarine.
One cup of herb tea after the meal, preferably peppermint, rosehip or camomile. 'Bambu' coffee may be used as an alternative.

Lunch
One plate of raw vegetables, especially carrots and beetroot, mixed with a dressing made from olive or sunflower oil together with a little lemon or celery juice.
Baked or steamed potatoes in their jackets may be taken with the vegetables.
For dessert, natural unflavoured yoghurt, sweetened with honey if necessary.

Dinner
Vegetable soup made with fresh, organically grown vegetables. These can be cooked in Plantaforce, a delicious vegetable concentrate from the Vogel range which is very easily digested. Use salt sparingly in this soup — a little Herbamare is more beneficial.
This can be followed by a little muesli, and then a fresh fruit salad. If there is a tendency to indigestion, do not combine these two.

General advice
Animal fat is prohibited. Use eggs sparingly. No white flour or white sugar (or products containing these), pork, sausages, bacon or ham. Cut down as much as possible on coffee, alcohol, nicotine and sweets.

4

Arteriosclerosis

THE WORD ARTERIOSCLEROSIS often brings a puzzled look to people's faces, but to put it in a nutshell it describes a condition of degeneration, when the inner walls of the arteries harden, mostly because of old age. It is frequently accompanied by high blood pressure.

Arteriosclerosis used to be nearly always associated with elderly people, but latterly, to my surprise, I have come across more and more younger people with similar complaints. Again, I fear that this trend could well be attributed to poor dietary management.

When people have consulted me about such problems I have been pleasantly surprised by the excellent results obtained after the patients have used oil of evening primrose and garlic capsules. I have also often recommended the extract of wild leeks, a remedy from the Bioforce range. In addition, although it may sound strange, someone who suffers from arteriosclerosis should always carry some dried currants or raisins, because chewing these at intervals during the day often proves beneficial.

The long-standing naturopathic approach to the treatment of arteriosclerosis, in order to restore the elasticity of the blood vessels, is dependent on how receptive a patient is to dietary changes. The naturopathic approach is often supported by herbal remedies and patients generally respond well.

There is no doubt that arteriosclerosis is caused by a process of degeneration. The progressive hardening of the arteries will result in a more sluggish movement of the blood through the body and therefore the toxic waste will not be properly disposed of. Hence an insufficient amount of oxygen will be transported through the body by the bloodstream which, in turn, will inevitably lead to further problems.

Mankind is affected by numerous influences outwith his control in the present environment, for example the effects of pollution, with the result that cardiovascular diseases are on the increase and are costing the taxpayer millions of pounds every year. However, we cannot place all the blame on outside influences because in many cases we take good health for granted and neglect to take proper care of our bodies. On the whole we eat too much animal protein and show a total disregard for ensuring a sensible balance in our diet. In this way we often introduce dangerous amounts of cholesterol and fats into our system. We carelessly continue to use saturated products, excess sugar and salt, thereby placing undue stress on the cardiovascular system and inviting a condition called lipotoxaemia, in which the blood contains excessive levels of fats and cholesterol.

How can we counter the increased viscosity of the blood and the decrease in oxygen? Regular exercise in the fresh air will certainly help to reduce the blood viscosity and thus the blood pressure, cholesterol and glucose levels. Arteriosclerosis, like all degenerative diseases, can be alleviated and sometimes even reversed if there is a reduction or elimination in the level of cholesterol triglyceride. Emotions, fears and anxieties can also be adverse influences on clogged and obstructed arteries and any reduction in these mental stresses will be useful. However, let me warn you that unless a diet that is low in cholesterol and sugar and lower in protein is adhered to, we cannot expect to reverse arteriosclerosis.

The Family Heart Association has supplied me with some very interesting reading material and statistics, some of which I refer to below, and I urge the reader to pay attention to these facts, as they cannot fail to impress. I would recommend anyone who suffers from heart problems, or is closely associated with someone in this category, to become a member of the Family Heart Association. The Association will be pleased to obtain your support and will supply any relevant information on request.

A high proportion of people who suffer coronaries at a young age or many family members with coronary heart disease have inherited conditions which cause high levels of fats (or lipids) in the blood. This type of condition is called hyperlipidaemia. These inherited conditions affect at least one in 300 people and result in a particularly high risk for coronary heart disease, but they are rarely diagnosed.

The Family Heart Association aims to:

1. increase awareness amongst the medical profession and the public about the familial hyperlipidaemias and of the need for a high-risk strategy for coronary prevention;
2. inform and support those affected;
3. encourage further research into the cause and treatment of the familial hyperlipidaemias.

The Association has stimulated and provided the background information for a number of television programmes, national and local radio programmes and newspaper articles throughout the country. Posters have been distributed to health centres and other public places, for example libraries. Printed booklets focusing on the possibilities of prevention are made available to doctors and members of the public and have been publicised at large medical conferences. So, you can see that it performs a very worthwhile task and is therefore worthy of your support.

One can imagine that coronary heart disease and arteriosclerosis are closely linked. It is claimed that a quarter of all deaths, and more than half the deaths of males in the 45-64 age group are due to heart disease. Hyperlipidaemia is an increasing problem and the result of an increase in the low density of lipoprotein which is the principal carrier protein for the transport of cholesterol in the bloodstream. Fortunately, there are a lot of ways that this condition can be kept at bay and my aim is to try and help you to find a way to reverse the process.

I remember one gentleman who had just turned sixty when he was diagnosed as an arteriosclerotic. He had recently retired from a demanding job and he was not inclined to give up his little "extras" in life, such as his daily tipple and his cigarettes. He felt that he was entitled to these little extravagances as they were part and parcel of the comfortable retirement he had been looking forward to. He told me that to keep his daughter happy he had followed her advice to take some vitamin E supplements and he imagined that he was feeling somewhat better as a result. He wondered if it was psychosomatic. Did he feel better because he expected to or was he really responding to the vitamin supplement? That was a loaded question to have put to you and therefore I asked him if he had ever heard of the saying "Man is what he eats".

When the improvement seemed to last and actually to increase, he began to wonder if it might be altogether more sensible if he gave up smoking and drinking. This was after quite some time, however, because he kept insisting that those little extras kept him happy. During one of our discussions I reminded him about his initial reaction to the benefits of vitamin supplements and how he himself had provided the proof for those claims. I tried to explain about the density of lipoproteins, the main carriers of cholesterol in the bloodstream, which increases the risk of arteriosclerosis. I told him about oxidation, low-density lipoproteins, so important as a chain-breaking anti-oxidant for which vitamin E is so necessary. It was probably this vitamin supplement that had supplied a shock to his system that had been geared to high fat levels because of his diet and these anti-oxidants might well have been the cause that his condition had been reversed to a certain degree. He became fascinated with the subject.

He then told me about the problems he experienced while walking. He claimed that after walking for only a short distance he would experience bad pains in his legs and would soon find himself out of breath. Eventually, he decided to stop smoking and drinking and to follow a course of treatment. He agreed to adjust his diet, continue with the vitamin supplements and to receive a course of Vasolastine injections as part of an enzyme therapy.

I have worked with this enzyme therapy for many years and I have seen amazing improvements in patients just like this gentleman. Therefore I was more than happy to advise him accordingly. I am pleased to say that he overcame his problems completely and as a sprightly elderly citizen he was able to enjoy his retirement despite having given up his few indulgences. He had previously regarded these as being essential to an enjoyable life, but had come to realise that without good health they were of little relevance.

I would like now to go into a little more detail on the

subject of the enzyme preparation Vasolastine. As I mentioned earlier, I have worked with this preparation for many years now and I have always been delighted with the results. To give you an indication of its effectiveness I quote a section from a report published by the International Journal for Research and Investigation on Atherosclerosis and Related Diseases in June 1982:

1. An enzyme preparation, Vasolastine, administered intramuscularly, to a group of elderly subjects reduced fasting plasma cholesterol and triglyceride levels by amounts which were proportional to their initial concentration.

2. Triglyceride levels three hours after a fat-rich meal are also directly dependent on the initial fasting level. This relationship is lowered significantly after twenty-five days of Vasolastine treatment.

3. Observations taken in conjunction with the results of in vitro studies confirm that Vasolastine acts synergistically with endogenous lipoprotein lipase.

Despite the diversity of theories advanced to elucidate the aetiology of atherosclerosis (another term for arteriosclerosis), it is widely accepted that the metabolism of the various lipoproteins assumes a vital role, since changing levels of individual lipoproteins control the amount of cholesterol carried in the plasma and thereby determine its availability for deposition in vascular tissue. Because of this, there is considerable interest in the role of lipoprotein lipase, the enzyme which controls the level of circulating lipoproteins following the ingestion of lipid.

The amount of lipid in the plasma depends on its rate of entry into the circulation from the gut via the lymph and the liver and on the rate of its removal by storage and oxidative metabolism.

Dietary cholesterol and triglycerides are transported in the plasma in the form of chylomicrons and very low density lipoproteins and postprandial triglyceridaemia result from an increase in these plasma constituents due to disturbances of the normal balance of intake and metabolism. Restoration of the balance would, in the first instance, depend on the enhancement of lipoprotein activity in the plasma.

It was demonstrated that one of the effects of prolonged intramuscular injection of the enzyme preparation Vasolastine was to lower the peak value for circulating lipids which occurs three to four hours after a fatty meal. The turbidity of the plasma was measured as an indication of the changing chylomicron count. It has already been shown that Vasolastine can materially affect plasma cholesterol levels in elderly subjects. The object of the present study is therefore to investigate the action of this preparation on the triglyceride components of alimentary lipaemia in an attempt to determine whether the preparation also acts synergistically with lipoprotein lipase in vivo.

Since the height of the plasma triglyceride peak which follows a fatty meal is related to (a) the rate of fat absorption and (b) the activity of the enzyme lipoprotein lipase (LPL), such a lowering of the peak value must imply that Vasolastine affects one of these factors. Marked changes in the passage of lipid across the intestinal mucosa might be affected by an enzyme preparation administered intramuscularly, but the most likely point of action would appear to be in the field of lipoprotein lipase activity.

Vasolastine could therefore: (a) contain LPL and hence enhance the plasma LPL concentration; (b) activate LPL by combining with it in lipolytic activity; (c) activate LPL by removing the products of reaction of this enzyme, e.g. by oxidation of free fatty acids or other metabolic reactions.

On the same subject of Vasolastine I read an interesting report on a pilot study performed by David A. Hall, Department of Medicine at the University of Leeds, and Roger Cox and Jenny Spanswick from the Netheredge

Hospital, Sheffield. A brief resumé of this report is as follows:

A randomised controlled double-blind trial of the lipolytic enzyme preparation Vasolastine in the treatment of certain manifestations atherosclerosis was conducted on sixty-two consecutively admitted elderly patients. The Vasolastine treated patients showed:

1. statistically significant improvements in several important clinical and biochemical parameters;

2. a statistically significant negative correlation between the change in total serum cholesterol and the pre-treatment level of this parameter;

3. That cholesterol bound to high density lipoprotein was unaffected by the treatment.

From the two latter points it may be deduced that the Vasolastine may be ascribed a therapeutic role in the treatment of type IIb lipoproteinaemias in patients of this age group.

Atherosclerosis causes, directly or indirectly, more than 40 per cent of deaths in western society. It is also responsible for some of the underlying pathologies associated with many symptoms of ageing. A geriatric population is therefore likely to have a high incidence of the various manifestations of this disease process. A pilot study investigating the influence of the enzyme-based preparation Vasolastine on severely ischaemic limbs was conducted in this unit and this encouraged us to make a more detailed examination of the product.

The manufacturers claim that Vasolastine favourably affects the atherosclerotic process. This claim is supported by various animal studies which show that it is capable of reversing severe atherosclerotic plaques in rabbits and rats and of mobilising lipid from their livers. Human studies have shown that the preparation can also affect plasma cholesterol levels and can reduce alimentary lipaemia following a fatty meal. Various other workers have reported functional improvements following its administration.

From these extracts you will appreciate how valuable enzyme therapy can be. in treating the conditions we are dealing with in this book.

I would like now to come back briefly to the subject of vitamin supplements. I have already pointed out the importance of vitamin E, but it is also valuable to know that oil of evening primrose taken in combination with vitamin E has proved very helpful. The same applies to the remedy Arterioforce, also mentioned earlier, as well as another Vogel remedy called *Vinca minor*. The latter is a fresh herb preparation used to treat disturbances in cerebral circulation and its consequences, such as lack of concentration and weakness of memory, as well as headaches, dizziness, noise in the ears, and difficulties in being able to adapt and in communication. These remedies may not work overnight but it should be remembered that arteriosclerosis is a slowly progressive condition that encroaches quietly, often without indications or symptoms becoming obvious until a relatively advanced stage has been reached. The more the arteries narrow the more likely it is that problems will arise.

In order to prevent coronary heart disease, it is essential to take steps to control arteriosclerosis. There are methods that allow us to do so and sometimes the condition can indeed be reversed. To this end a low cholesterol diet is essential and sometimes I even advise people to follow a macrobiotic diet for a while. More specialised diets can be found in later chapters on the relevant subjects.

I have had extremely encouraging feedback from arterio-sclerotics after they had decided to take the bull by the horns and work positively towards improving their health. It may take some initial effort to adjust to a new regime, but the necessary changes need not be too drastic. Never forget that is is your own health that is at stake and the effort will therefore be more worthwhile. Remember, too, that it is the *quality* of the food we consume that provides the improvement and never the *quantity*.

Draw up a plan and remember that the body will repay you with better health for the effort you make. We know that arteriosclerosis is not a new problem; nevertheless, it is worrying to see its rate of increase. In the field of naturopathy we have been advising patients for years that paying due attention to their diet is part of the solution for vascular disorders. It is encouraging to learn that many of our orthodox colleagues are now also advising arteriosclerotic patients with a high cholesterol level of the benefits of eating porridge.

The term atheroma, which is derived from the Greek word for porridge, was first used in 1904 when Morchand initiated the term atherosclerosis, a different name for arteriosclerosis. It is interesting to see that both names point to a process that involves the arteries, in one way or another, depositing fats.

On my return from a recent trip to India where in a short spell of time I had seen more than 1,000 patients, I was pondering on the fact that vascular diseases did not appear to be very common there. I do not doubt, however, that this respite will be short-lived when I think of the so-called "civilised" food products that are being imported into that country; for by doing so I am convinced that they are also importing some of our western health problems.

Take a lesson from Nature: *We are born from Nature, we belong to Nature and we should obey the laws of Nature.*

5

Cholesterol

THE YOUNG DOCTOR sitting opposite me looked twice at the file on her desk and said that she could not believe her eyes. "How in the world is it possible that you have a cholesterol reading of nearly eight?" I have to admit that the results came as quite a shock to me too and I suggested that she might want to take another test. The doctor was certain, however, that the results were valid. She asked me about my diet and whether I drank or smoked. I could reassure her on all three points. She then asked if I took porridge for breakfast and because I am well aware how good this is for one's general health and especially for one's cholesterol level, I again confirmed that I did. She also wanted to know if I ate many eggs and here again I could reassure her — a maximum of two eggs a week. I explained that my diet largely consisted of cereals, fresh fruit and vegetables and yoghurt and that, where possible, I tried to minimise my intake of animal fats and sugars. What, then, could be the reason for the high cholesterol level?

Having been in practice myself for more than thirty years, I knew what the doctor was looking for. On hindsight I could certainly think of one or two reasons why my cholesterol level was so much higher than it ought to have been and so I told her that at the time the test was taken I had been under considerable stress. I had been required to attend several formal dinners and because of lack of time I had not been able to take any exercise. On average I spend up to ninety hours a week in treatment rooms with patients, under artificial light, etc. The reading served the purpose of making me realise that I would have to be stricter with myself and start to practise what I preached.

I decided to pay strict attention to my diet and exercise regime for the next month or so. I also made up my mind to somehow find the time to take a walk for at least half an hour every day, as well as to take more time to wind down and meditate again. Thankfully, I have a sound and healthy immune system; that, together with the measures mentioned above, helped to bring down my cholesterol level quite quickly. I also made it part of my routine to eat some grapes every day, remembering to thoroughly chew the pips. Every day I took one oral chelation tablet and I sprinkled some Sojaforce on my breakfast porridge. Sojaforce is a food supplement which contains natural vitamin E in a form that is easily absorbed by the body and is necessary for the function of the muscles and gonads. The instantly soluble granules of high quality protein obtained from milk, wheatgerm and soya bean taste especially good dissolved in orange juice or milk, or even just sprinkled on cereal, and are easily digested. Before the month was out my cholesterol level was back to what it should have been in the first place.

Now let us look at what cholesterol really is, apart from a word that has recently become quite fashionable. In the blood is a lipid fraction in the triglycerol and free fatty acids which includes cholesterol, a highly important fat which is also called phospholipid and is similar to lecithin or certain vitamins or hormones. Cholesterol is not soluble in water and therefore in the blood plasma these lipids remain suspended in the blood after they have been formed into fat proteins called lipoproteins. Our body then makes an outer shell to the water soluble proteins in which the triglycerides, cholesterol and other lipids are contained. These are formed into little particles, sometimes called "balls". They are suspended in the blood plasma as they are in the water soluble coat of protein. These little balls are compressed in high density or even extremely high density lipoproteins. They also contain a far higher than average amount of triglycerides and cholesterol and are much heavier than water.

Although we are often led to believe that cholesterol is the main factor contributing to cardiovascular conditions, this is not completely true. Conditions such as strokes, angina, kidney failure or heart attacks are generally the result of a very gradual process during which the cholesterol and fats progressively become deposited among the normal cells. The arteries and the muscle layer rely on the efficient transportation of oxygen in the bloodstream. High levels of fats and cholesterol have to be absorbed within the artery wall and if this process is too extreme then there is the danger that the cells of the artery will burst. If this happens, our innate healing capacity will probably come to the rescue and restore the damaged area; new cells will be formed together with more fibrous tissue, creating a hardened plaque in the artery wall which may restrict the flow of blood. This plaque is the scar tissue.

Other conditions may cause the artery to lose its elasticity and certain deposits will form themselves into particles which might cause much more serious problems. Eventually, these little plaques on the inner wall of the artery will interfere with the blood flow and it is very often the loose particles that can cause disastrous effects, sometimes even fatality. The existence of such particles within the artery cannot be ignored and therefore it is important to realise how they come into existence.

Without doubt nicotine, alcohol, stress and dietary mismanagement must be considered major contributory factors. Even by introducing a low-cholesterol diet we cannot take it for granted that this process of plaque formation, or calcification, can be completely forestalled or reversed. Sometimes patients ask me if all veins contain cholesterol. Yes, certainly, cholesterol is present in all veins and arteries, but plaque formation only takes place in the arteries.

Cholesterol is a very slippery substance that usually slips and slides through the blood vessels. This slippery mass is definitely not harmless, but it does not represent as great a cause for concern as the little particles. Cholesterol is also a vital substance and is present in every cell in the body; it is a component of bile and of hormones and it also helps in the manufacture of vitamin D under the skin. In view of the fact that it is a necessary substance, what we are concerned with is ways in which to control cholesterol, not to eliminate it.

In cases of an artery blockage the coronary bypass operation has often proved to be very successful. Nevertheless, this does not solve the problem completely. Such a bypass operation can be performed on the major blood vessels but it is hardly conclusive if there are circulatory problems.

In a report in the *British Medical Journal* of November 1985 I read that tests had concluded that of a sample of 312 patients who had undergone coronary artery bypass surgery 190, that is 61 per cent, had experienced postoperational neurological problems. Most of the patients — 72 per cent — were not seriously disabled, but fifteen suffered strokes, ten failed to regain consciousness and twenty-five developed blurred vision or some other form of deterioration of their eyesight. Although we have reason to be grateful for the science that enables surgeons to perform bypass operations, the onus lies with each individual to prevent as much as possible the necessity for such drastic surgery.

A high proportion of cholesterol in the tissue, in the brain or in the spinal cord, is also involved in the manufacture of hormones and the cholesterol that circulates in the bloodstream, also called a serum cholesterol. This in part accounts for the lipoproteins, of which there are several kinds, such as Alpha, Beta and pre-Beta. Involvement of this part of the cholesterol in the nervous system is responsible for a normal process and its effectiveness is again subject to our dietary management.

The way in which dietary cholesterol enters the bloodstream is clearly defined in the book *The Liver, the Regulator of Your Health*, written by Dr Vogel. The three substances that the liver clearly disagrees with are animal fats, nicotine and alcohol. In many cases this wonderful laboratory becomes so overloaded with these substances that it becomes unable to cope. The liver's main task is to receive the nutrients via the intestines and, if necessary, store them so that the correct balance is maintained in the body. Although the body is capable of making its own cholesterol, it is nevertheless dependent on the cholesterol obtained from our food. It is here that common sense becomes so essential. The body is only able to handle a certain quantity of cholesterol. Let us take, for instance, polyunsaturated fats: these can have the effect of high concentrations via the liver and gallbladder joining up to form cholesterol which is then crystallised to make gallstones. It is obvious that fit people will be able to handle dietary cholesterol much better than people who have health problems, so again it is important to take care to abide by the dietary rules.

With a little extra thought and consideration, this need not be so difficult, because relatively few foods actually contain cholesterol. In general, foods from an animal origin, such as meat, eggs, chicken and dairy produce, are high in protein as well as cholesterol. It is also well known that liver and certain shellfish have a high cholesterol content. It is advisable to introduce some unrefined carbohydrates into the diet as this will help to maintain our digestive system and our ability to absorb the food in good order. Some degree of dietary adjustment is often required in order to reduce the levels of blood cholesterol in the arteries and the body tissues. The most important guidelines, therefore, concern the low cholesterol diet mentioned in the previous chapter, as well as paying serious consideration to the use of nicotine and alcohol and keeping careful check on the stress factor. There are, however, other means that can be used in the battle to reduce a cholesterol level that is too high.

Along with diet, exercise deserves our attention, because regular exercise is a preventative measure; it stimulates all the internal organs, helps us to sleep and lowers the cholesterol level. Why not decide to go for a good swim two or three times a week, or for a long walk or bicycle ride. There is a whole range of suitable activities which will not place us under undue pressure even if we are not quite so young anymore. It is an undeniable fact that a fit sportsperson rarely experiences cholesterol-related problems.

Let us not forget about the benefits of vitamins, minerals and trace elements. For instance, it has been shown that vitamin C is helpful to people with high blood pressure as it eases the pressure on the arteries. Calcium can also do the same thing. Vitamin B_6 is beneficial in the metabolism of essential fatty acids and is therefore relevant in the maintenance of a healthy circulation. Vitamin E, as we have seen, is also considered to reduce the level of cholesterol. Many recent tests have concluded that in what we consider to be a "civilised diet" the intake of certain vitamins, minerals and trace elements is too low. When we add to these nutritional factors the influence of stress and pollution we have a serious combination of factors that leads to poor circulation, strokes, heart attacks and, not infrequently, even death. This realisation has prompted certain American and Canadian scientists to develop a multiple nutritional formula and make it available as a supplement that is now referred to as chelation therapy.

What exactly is chelation therapy? It was first introduced in 1948 in the United States, containing several vitamins, minerals and trace elements, to combat the effects of lead poisoning. However, in trials it was discovered that it also served to lower the cholesterol level and even emulsify or dissolve the loose particles present in the arteries. Chelation therapy is also effective in widening the narrowed arteries. Much research has been undertaken to try to substantiate or refute such claims, but unfortunately the controversy on the benefits of chelation therapy still continues. For me, however, the proof can be found in the enthusiastic testimonies of patients who have used this therapy — and their testimonies are virtually unanimous in their praise. Results such as these cannot be disputed.

Chelation therapy is actually a nutritional remedy and an effective combination of chelating nutrients obtained from natural sources. It can be administered by injection, but if preferred oral chelation is available. No adverse side-effects have been reported and it appears that chelation therapy can effect a reversal of the hardening of the arteries and that instead the bones and teeth are strengthened.

Obviously, chelation therapy has attracted a great deal of interest. In recent years it has also captured the attention of the well-known health practitioner and Nobel

Prize winner Dr Linus Pauling, the great advocate of vitamin C, who has endorsed chelation therapy by saying: "I think it is an invaluable kind of treatment for many patients and as an alternative to therapy not just for the heart bypass patient but for patients with a variety of problems." I have noticed that it has become widely accepted that chelation therapy reduces toxic metal deposits, high blood pressure, blood cholesterol, calcium deposits and sometimes kidney stones and that it greatly improves the circulation, skin texture, liver function, hearing, vision and general well-being. So, all in all, it has given tremendous hope to people with cholesterol and other problems.

It is of course up to the individual to take action, as ultimately we are responsible for our own health. There is no single "miracle" ingredient available that will do the trick unsupported. Rather, it is the synergistic total of all ingredients working together and supporting each other. In my experience, the daily intake of each supplementary nutrient necessary to produce the vascular cleansing response are most effectively combined in the FLW formula, which is made as follows:

Vitamin A	25,000–50,000 IU
Vitamin E (d-alpha)	600–900 IU
Vitamin C	3,000–6,000 mg
Vitamin B_1	200–270 mg
Vitamin B_2 (riboflavin)	45–50 mg
Niacin	50–105 mg
Niacinamide	30–50 mg
Pantothenic Acid	250–500 mg
Vitamin B_6 (pyrodoxine)	150–225 mg
Folic acid	400–900 mcg
Vitamin B_{12} (cobalamin)	240–250 mcg
Biotin	75–100 mcg
Choline (bitartrate)	725–940 mg
Inositol	40–100 mg

Magnesium (oxide)	400–630 mg
Zinc (gluconate)	25–37 mg
Chromium (acetate)	195–250 mcg
Selenium (dioxide)	250–300 mcg

This is indeed an impressive formula and one that can be taken alongside other medication without adverse effects. The results will not be noticeable overnight, but one will gradually become aware of an improvement. This remarkable formula has also proved to be of great help in the treatment of other problems such as headaches, intestinal gas, nausea and diarrhoea. Moreover, no toxicity has been shown to result from its use.

Knowing that our drinking water has not been up to standard for quite some time now, because of chemical additives and pollution in general, I sometimes recommend the FLW chelation formula in cases where I suspect excess toxicity.

I remember one elderly gentleman who had struggled up the single outside step at the entrance to our clinic and then stood there pondering on how to cope with the three small steps inside the front door until a member of our staff came to his assistance. He told me that all his life he had been able to walk well. He was a retired farmer and was used to walking round his fields without any problem whatsoever. It did not take long to convince him that I might be able to help him, because he was very upset by the loss of his independence caused by his inability to move about unaided. I considered him an excellent candidate for chelation therapy, but wanted to ease him into it, partly in view of his advanced age. I advised him to take one tablet of FLW and one tablet of Chelating Mega Mineral Complex from Nature's Best. The results were amazing: three weeks later he returned to the clinic with a big grin on his face to tell me that his legs felt much stronger and that the heaviness he experienced was diminishing. Another six weeks later he claimed proudly that once again he was able to walk without a stick. Such is the encouraging feedback I receive when I have decided to prescribe a remedy that, unfortunately, still causes so much controversy. I still see this old gentleman and he is perfectly happy and never fails to sing the praises of this remedy because it has given him a new lease of life.

Before continuing I would like to tell you a little more about the remedy I have just mentioned — Chelating Mega Mineral Complex. This is a potent formula of essential minerals in a hypo-allergenic base containing chromium and selenium. It is based on a vegetarian formulation that contains mega potencies of all the essential minerals, as follows:

Calcium (as carbonate and phosphate)	1,000 mg
Magnesium (as oxide)	500 mg
Phosphorus (as calcium phosphate)	200 mg
Potassium (amino acid complex)	99 mg
Zinc (as gluconate)	50 mg
Iron (as fumarate)	27 mg
Manganese (as gluconate)	10 mg
Iodine (as potassium iodide)	225 mcg
21 amino acid mix	450 mg

Let us now briefly sum up what we have learned about the cholesterol problem. This fatty substance is often referred to as aemia, which means that it is in the blood. People with high blood cholesterol are more prone to coronary heart disease. Familial hypercholesterolaemia is the term used when high blood cholesterol is inherited and passed from one generation to the next. I have not mentioned this illness before, but this is something that can be determined fairly easily and it may be helpful to know whether or not one might be susceptible to this condition. It can be apparent through swellings in the tendons and/or on the backs of the hands or ankles, indicating a build-up of cholesterol there. Another common symptom of familial hypercholesterolaemia is a creamy white adge in part of the eye, especially in younger people under the age of forty. Also, yellow lumps or streaks of fats in the skin close to the eyes could well indicate a tendency to high blood cholesterol among close relatives.

If such signs are noticed, you would be wise not to let the matter rest but to pursue it further and arrange to undergo a cholesterol test. If the diagnosis is familial hypercholesterolaemia, you would do well to use the relatively new remedy called Silica, which is marvellous for just such conditions. Also remember that good quantities of silica can be obtained from oat bran, so you may consider including this as a regular feature of your dietary regime.

The use of essential fatty acids (EFAs) must be considered, to control the fats obtained from our diet, and these are important components of any well-balanced diet. We frequently hear about the benefits of oil of evening primrose or blackcurrant seed oil; these are very important supplements as they contain alphalinoleic acids, which encourage the manufacture of protective eicosapentaenoic acid and EFAs. A shortage of EFAs can lead to a whole range of metabolic problems and therefore they are clearly important for maintaining good health. In Chapter 11, where I will examine possible preventative measures in greater detail, I will provide more information on the use of EFAs and on their importance.

The remedies outlined below will help to reduce the cholesterol level, especially when combined with a well-balanced dietary regime. We must never forget that a diet rich in saturated fats has been identified as a serious risk factor with regard to coronary disease, so some guidelines that double as a means of preventing cholesterol build-up will be even more helpful.

—Make very sure that the use of butter and margarine is limited to the bare necessity.

—Use no more than three eggs a week.

—Take cottage cheese or low fat cheese instead of rich full fat cheeses.

—If eating meat, choose lean varieties, but it is preferable to follow a vegetarian diet. Never use pork in any form, that is bacon, ham, gammon, etc.

—Exclude all cooking fats such as lard, dripping or ordinary vegetable oil; if necessary, use sunflower oil, safflower oil, corn oil or soya oil, but even then only sparingly.

—Replace full fat cows' milk with skimmed milk or soya milk.

—Be careful with salt and sugar, as these represent health hazards.

—Restrict the use of convenience or pre-packed foods to the minimum.

—Take great care to avoid constipation and to keep the body weight down.

Do not forget that, like one's general health, a cholesterol problem is the individual's own responsibility as it is often self-inflicted through ignorance or lack of interest. Dr Albert Schweitzer, the great physician, showed great wisdom when he said that every patient carries within him his own physician. The doctor's job is merely to evoke that physician.

6

Strokes and Thrombosis

I ALWAYS HAVE great sympathy for the patient who comes to me for advice after having been the victim of a stroke. Mostly they are elderly, but sometimes they are still quite young, in which case the inability to perform tasks previously taken for granted is often even harder to bear. Whatever the circumstances, a great deal of understanding and patience is required. Anyone who has led an active life finds it very hard to have to accept that suddenly, after a stroke, they are not capable of doing the things they used to do without giving them a second thought.

Strange though it may seem, one of the characteristics of stroke patients appears to be that they all used to be active and energetic, then, suddenly, this is called to a halt. How can one cope with this and is there anything that can be done about it?

It is pointless to tell the stroke patient that he or she should have slowed down before the damage was done. The condition, by that stage, has revealed itself and that fact cannot be undone. Frequently, the use of the arms and legs is impaired and the patient has the resulting mental frustrations to cope with as well as the physical handicaps themselves. With the tendency for blood pressure irregularities already present, he or she is unlikely to help their own condition unless a positive decision is made to find out what can be done to improve the situation.

Stroke patients generally react well to the Vogel remedy Auroforce. This is a fresh herb preparation suitable for nervous heart complaints that are accompanied by feelings of anxiety and difficulty in breathing and also for conditions of low blood pressure caused by weak circulation. The remedy is composed of the following ingredients:

Crataegus oxyacantha	— hawthorn berry
Valeriana off.	— valerian
Cactus grandiflorus	— blooming cereus
Ilex aquifolium	— holly
Hyssopus off.	— hyssop

When taken in combination with an FLW tablet each night and morning, this remedy can be of great benefit to stroke patients.

What actually happens when one suffers a stroke? We have already seen how when the heart muscle does not receive the required blood supply for even a few minutes, the section of the muscle concerned will perish and scar tissue will eventually form. The extent of the damage is usually recognised with the aid of an electrocardiogram. The occurrence of a stroke is also referred to as an "infarct" or "infarction", that is an area of dead or dying tissue resulting from obstruction of the blood vessels that normally supply the part affected. An infarct need not necessarily take place in the heart muscle; it could equally well affect the brain, in which case paralysis will be the result. Facial paralysis might occur, or difficulty with speech, or a one-sided paralysis where, for example, the limbs on one side of the body are rendered powerless. If a clot becomes lodged in the pulmonary artery, between the heart and the lungs, this can be the cause of a sudden heart attack or a pulmonary embolism. A stroke is indeed quite serious as the effects are usually such that they cannot be totally reversed.

A stroke is a manifestation of a cardiovascular disease affecting the arteries supplying the brain. A partial blockage will not always result in the complete destruction of brain tissue as there will usually remain sufficient blood flow to keep the cells alive. An artery can withstand tremendous pressure, although when it does rupture there will be serious problems; this is referred to as a haemorrhage, when large quantities of blood escape from a blood vessel.

In our clinic in Scotland I have treated stroke patients for almost twenty years and it is a sad fact that there the incidence of strokes is the highest in the world. I have been able to follow the steady progress of many of my patients, but I have also studied a number of cases where no improvement was noticeable.

One of the most important factors is how the stroke patient adapts to the new lifestyle that he or she is forced to adopt. No good will come from frustration, although avoiding this is easier said than done. The lesson to be learned is that the stroke has taken place and the clock cannot be turned back and it is a case of positively deciding to do something about it. Often, the normal channels of physiotherapy are open to such patients, and they will soon become aware of their physical limitations. Then the time will have come to consider some natural remedies as a means of improving on these recognised limitations. If a nervous condition is involved, I can highly recommend the Vogel remedy Neuroforce, which is a restorative remedy for nervous

71

exhaustion. It helps to retain mental and physical capacity and prevents the loss of vitality and should be used during convalescence to counter overtiredness, general listless-ness and lack of appetite. The components of Neuroforce are as follows:

Calcium gluconate
Avena sativa trit.
Glutamic acid
Lecithin
Natrium phosphoricum
Radix Ginseng

Together with Neuroforce, in many cases I would suggest that a stroke patient also takes a multivitamin preparation as this will support the muscle tissue.

If medically advised that an anti-coagulant is necessary and the patient cannot take any more aspirin or any other painkiller, he or she might think about taking a natural anti-coagulant, which may help to slowly reduce the need for the drug that is less well tolerated. In his book *Nature — Your Guide to Healthy Living*, Dr Vogel writes about the properties of garden chervil, which is not to be confused with wild chervil. This is an excellent alternative remedy if an anti-coagulant is con-sidered essential. In Switzerland garden chervil has been used for such purposes for many years. It has a strong aromatic scent and is classified as an aromatic herb, but it also has medicinal properties. It can be finely chopped and sprinkled on salads and soups as it has a pleasant taste. This plant has the effect of thinning the blood and when there are fears of embolism or thrombosis, it is an extremely reliable supplement. However, chervil con-tains coumarin and must not be over-used. It is therefore not to be used indiscriminately, but can be taken safely on a daily basis for all kinds of nodular formation such as haemorrhoids or varicose veins. Taken together with a tablet of Kelpasan, which after a little while can be increased to two tablets taken first thing in the morning, chervil will be very beneficial. Kelpasan is made from pure sea algae from the Pacific Ocean, and contains a wealth of trace elements. It is a natural supplement for iodine deficiency and serves as a prophylaxis for goitre. Kelpasan stimulates the cell metabolism of the endocrine glands and increases mental and physical capacity. It can be safely used except in the case of thyroid dysfunction, when it is advisable to consult a medical practitioner instead.

When a stroke patient experiences no improvement to their physical limitations, some acupuncture treatment may be called for. In particular, the relatively few people who do not respond to, or tolerate, blood thinners, tranquillisers, blood-pressure-regulating drugs or sleeping tablets, seem to respond well to acupuncture treatment.

With longer-term manifestations we see more cardio-vascular blockages and perhaps more cardiac inability. The prevention of cardiac failure entails the preservation of all activities in a properly aligned bone structure. We should not forget that with any dislocation of a bone there will be a disturbance or a chain reaction on the entire structure. In this respect we see that acupuncture can fill a great gap.

Sometimes, auricular acupuncture may be selected to release tension or even pain, but several other forms of acupuncture can be used to reverse or correct such a situation. Using acupuncture, I have been able to help many a patient who had made no progress by other means. It is not unreasonable to expect a gradual improvement when one follows sound advice and takes care to reduce the influence of the contributory factors that have been outlined above.

Also after thrombosis there are many helpful ways to overcome the physical invalidity that usually results. Thrombosis can occur when the blood platelets show an increased tendency to gather together and in so doing a clotting process is initiated with a presence of high concentrations of cholesterol. For this condition, oil of evening primrose can be beneficial, together with vitamin E. Another excellent remedy to use is *Hamamelis virginiana* (witch hazel) and this remedy is especially suitable for veinous congestion and haemorrhoids, for dilation and inflammation of the veins, and for bleeding haemorrhoids and varicose veins. Also recommended is the homoeopathic potency of Lachesis D12, which is a very low potency of snake poison, to be taken together with Urticalcin. The latter is a homoeopathic calcium and silicic acid preparation for use where a lack of calcium is indicated. Urticalcin helps to build the bones and improves brittle nails and loss of hair. It can serve as a preventative measure when excessive amounts of acid are present in the body.

A simple self-help suggestion is to eat on alternative days a slice of wholewheat bread with rosehip jam, while on the other days the slice of wholewheat bread can be spread with a mixture of honey and Urticalcin. A thrombosis patient cannot go wrong by following this simple advice.

When a tendency to clotting is recognised, one must aim to control thrombus formation and keep the arteries in check in order to maintain a balance of thrombolytic prostaglandin, which is also called prostacycline. Through experience I have come to the conclusion that with such clot-forming problems another remedy can be very helpful. This is a combination remedy, marketed under my own name in the range of Nature's Gift remedies and it has oil of evening primrose, blackcurrant seed oil, royal jelly, scotiaberry and vitamin E as its ingredients.

Coronary thrombosis patients are often subject to fluctuating emotional influences. Lack of energy and movement are common place and so the end result could well be an increase in circulatory complaints. If the blood circulation is poor, feelings of depression are often reported. This can sometimes be overcome by simple exercises, whereas maintaining a negative attitude will often cause the patients to be their worst enemy. If you fall into this category, do an exercise in some mental research and ask yourself some pertinent questions, such as:

—Do I feel in harmony with my body, my head, my feelings, my heart?
—Do I do things half-heartedly?
—Do I often feel aggressive or in conflict with things that are happening?
—Can I discuss my problem with others, or do I feel that the problem is mine alone and I have to live with it without burdening others with it?

The answers to these questions will have a significant bearing on your chance of recovery, because they will be indicative of your mental attitude. Give your emotions room to breathe. Perhaps you might try asking yourself a question my mother sometimes asked me when I was young — and I am quite sure that my mother was not the only parent who asked her child such a question when the child was faced with a dilemma. The question was: "Why don't you listen to the voice in your heart?"

7

Blood Circulation

IT IS NO EXAGGERATION to say that blood is a vital ingredient of life. It performs an admirable task in that it transports oxygen and nutrition to all the cells and organs in the body, ultimately through to the lungs and kidneys, and it also disposes of waste matter from the excretory organs. This red liquid also distributes vitamins, minerals, trace elements, antibodies and coagulating agents throughout the body. Because of the many adverse influences we encounter today, it is considered quite an achievement if we manage to keep our blood clear of invaders, for example viruses, which can be the cause of all kinds of illness and disease, some of them very hard to combat once they have taken hold.

Actually, if it were not for the red blood cells this wonderful liquid would really be transparent yellow or off-white in colour. At birth we have approximately half a pint of blood and as an adult this will have increased to between eight and ten pints, which accounts for about 10 per cent of our body weight. When we donate blood, the body will voluntarily produce more blood to make up the difference and bring its volume back to the same level as before the blood was extracted.

As stated above, the red colour of the blood is due to the red blood cells, also called erythrocytes. These contain haemoglobin, which is in the red colouring matter of the red blood corpuscles. Each drop of blood travels more than three kilometres a day, and there is constant and dynamic change in these red blood cells which have such an important role to play. Next to the red blood cells we have the white blood cells, called leukocytes. These are colourless and of irregular shape. It is said that one cubic millimetre of healthy blood from an adult contains from 5,000 to 9,000 leukocytes. Among these white blood cells we can recognise three different cell types: the granulocytes, the lymphocytes and the monocytes. The lymphocytes come from the lymph system and have a clearly defined origin, whilst it is still not completely known what the origin of the monocytes is. The granulocytes are mostly contained in the tissues. The blood platelets, which are called thrombocytes, form the smallest cell components of the blood. They fill the very important role of blood-coagulating agents. Taken together, these cells contribute to a system that involves a process no factory on earth is capable of.

Blood plasma contains many components, such as sugars, fats, vitamins, minerals, trace elements and also gammaglobulin, a protein which is important for the immune system. In the protein plasma, a chemical reaction of vital importance takes place and the most important job it performs is to bind oxygen into oxyhaemoglobin. Haemoglobin carries oxygen from the lungs to the tissues and it transports carbon dioxide from the tissues to the lungs. The connection between haemoglobin and carboxy-haemoglobin is extremely important in a healthy blood count.

Good circulation of this primitively explained process is essential and blood circulatory problems will occur if the normal circulation of this wonder liquid is somehow interfered with. All kinds of problems can occur when adverse influences are allowed the chance to gain strength. These include aggregation of the red blood cells, reduced oxygen pick-up, as well as increased blood viscosity, inability of the capillaries to receive the red blood cells, and possibly oedema, arteriosclerosis and quite a few more.

We often find that the blood circulation suffers under the influence of a toxic high viscosity. This may indeed cause serious problems as the circulation will be geared up to counteract such irregularities and this could well lead to other problems.

An elderly female patient asked me the other day if I believed that blood was merely a chemical substance or if indeed it had anything to do with our emotional or spiritual life. I told her that in the oldest book of the world, in the Bible, it is said that "the soul is in the blood". The mysterious actions that take place in the blood are something very special and it is largely beyond human comprehension how exactly the blood works and what the influencing factors are. You will know the saying that you are as old as you feel, but I have also heard it put as follows: "You are as old as your blood circulation."

You would readily agree that our circulatory system merits our fullest support if you learned that during a time spell of twenty-four hours eleven tons of blood are pumped through the body. Any small irregularity has an effect on the smooth circulation of the blood.

Having made this statement on the blood circulatory system, I will tell you about a young man who came to see me in a quite off-hand fashion. I recognised in him all the symptoms of Raynaud's disease, but he did not appear to be unduly worried. Raynaud's disease is a condition of recurring vascular spasms of the extremities, caused by ischaemia in the limbs. Because of constriction of the blood vessels the blood supply to an organ or tissue cannot pass unhindered and the disease manifests itself mostly in the fingers and toes. These outer extremities will turn white and occasionally gangrene can set in.

When I tried to tell this young man about this medical condition he brusquely replied that he had learned to live with it and mostly it hardly bothered him. In the same breath, however, he mumbled that lately he had been feeling considerably more discomfort, but he was sure that this would pass. He was utterly shocked when I warned him that the next stage could well be gangrene. Already he had reached the stage of painful ulcers, without having been aware of the further deterioration that had taken place. He then wholeheartedly agreed that he would follow my advice if I could suggest remedial treatment. He was the kind of person who took an "all or nothing" approach. Once he had been convinced that something ought to be done about his condition he really became determined that only his best would be good enough.

Fortunately, he responded very well to one of Dr Vogel's remedies called Petasan — a herbal remedy which has as its main ingredient *Viscum album*, or mistletoe. Petasan is often prescribed for spastic conditions, weak circulation, the initial period after infectious illnesses and for cases of nutritional deficiencies. Together with Petasan, he agreed to take a vitamin E supplement and to receive twice weekly injections of the Vasolastine enzyme. This young man very soon reported that he was making significant progress and this encouraged him sufficiently to strictly adhere to the treatment. Where previously he had decided to let things slide and learn to live with his symptoms, he now had turned over a new leaf. Having been shocked into taking the first step, he had become determined to go all the way towards a full recovery.

This case was slightly reminiscent of that of an elderly female patient who stated from the first that she had never used any medicine or remedies in the past and was not about to start now. She was, however, a great believer in the old form of medicine called hydrotherapy. She was therefore interested when I told her about a fairly harsh remedy which in our clinic is referred to as "the cold dip". This is a version of hydrotherapy that I learned about in the Far East and it served this elderly lady very well, bringing about a significant improvement in her circulatory system. You may think that this method is too simple to expect any results, but let me assure you that when the benefits are plain to see, you will agree that treatments need not always be expensive to be beneficial.

The cold dip exercise has to be done faithfully every morning on getting up and each evening on retiring. Place a basin of cold water at the side of the bed, together with a towel. Immediately on getting up in the morning, place both feet into the water. Count to ten and remove the feet from the water and place them on the towel, to be dabbed dry. Exercise the toes as if trying to pick up a marble. Repeat this sequence 10–30 times. The same procedure should be carried out before retiring at night. You will find that your feet will be as warm as toast when you go to bed. The important thing to remember with this exercise is that it should be done for a minimum of sixty days in order to obtain its full benefits.

After this lady had begun to improve somewhat, I spoke to her about diet and casually mentioned the advantage of taking a vitamin supplement. Although initially she did not appear very eager, she agreed to take vitamin E. I explained to her that because of her impaired muscular co-ordination and reflexes there was a loss of sensation in the peripheral nerves that I was sure vitamin E would help to overcome. This recommendation is applicable to all age groups, because I have seen the results of tests involving children who had deficiencies in vitamin E which show that this can easily result in neurological problems and loss of muscle co-ordination or tendon reflexes.

Nature's Best produces a supplement called Imuno-Strength, which is compiled according to my own formula. The name Imuno-Strength speaks for itself: a remedy to boost our immune response. It is described as a multi-nutritional vitamin and mineral formula because it encourages the immune system to deal with viruses, bacteria and toxins before they become established in the bloodstream. Today's world is full of challenges to our defence mechanism and these challenges include environmental pollution by potentially toxic chemicals. In these circumstances, it makes sense to help protect the integrity of our immune system by safeguarding our nutrition. So, as well as carefully selected amounts of vitamins and minerals known to be needed for the proper functioning of the immune system, Imuno-Strength contains the herbs, devil's claw and echinacea. I have also insisted that Imuno-Strength include 15 mg of thymus gland concentrate, as the T-cells of the immune system have their base in the thymus. Imuno-Strength acts as an anti-oxidant and will help when gradual deterioration is being caused by excessive oxidation.

From an interesting report I read recently I learned that vitamin E can also help to arrest the abnormalities in the red blood cells of new-born babies affected by sickle cell anaemia, as vitamin E is known to protect the red cell membranes by blocking the peroxidation process and stabilising the membrane layer. It seems that sickle cell disease is due to sickle-haemoglobin and in some irreversible sickle cells there is a lower plasma of vitamin E levels.

If only our food contained suffcient vitamins, minerals and trace elements, then there would be fewer health problems. Whatever the reasons are, however, vitamin deficiency is indeed a very real problem nowadays, but one that can often be dealt with by a supplementary formula. I must stress that if larger dosages of vitamins are being considered, then one should first seek the advice of a medical practitioner. Mostly I consider 500–600 IU of vitamin E to be sufficient, especially when this is taken over a considerable period.

In connection with the blood circulation, it is worth pointing out the benefits of physical exercise. Outdoor exercise must be considered to be one of the best ways to improve circulatory problems. Also remember hydrotherapy — why not try the cold dip that I mentioned earlier (see page 80). Taking alternate hot and cold sitzbaths is another effective form of hydrotherapy.

It is encouraging to see that Nature offers us a variety of remedies, some of which are ideally suited for the treatment of circulatory problems. I shall never forget my first year in Scotland. I had just moved with my family from the Netherlands and not for one moment had I dared to hope that the clinic I intended to establish in Scotland would develop as quickly as it did. At that time I had not yet had the opportunity to import a wide variety of remedies from Switzerland, but I had been able to obtain a supply of the excellent remedy called Hyperisan. I was astonished by the number of people I managed to help in those early days, largely thanks to this single remedy. I soon learned that in the north of Scotland and on the islands the older generation especially were well aware of the healing properties of St John's wort (*Hypericum perforatum*), which is the principal ingredient of the remedy Hyperisan. *Hypericum* in combination with the other ingredients of *Achillea millefolium* (yarrow), *Aesculus hippocastanum* (horse chestnut) and *Arnica montana e radix* (arnica herb and root) must rate as one of the finest herbal remedies available. In my book *Traditional Home and Herbal Remedies*, I have written in greater detail about this remedy and its applications for a diverse range of problems.

Blood circulatory disorders are often accompanied by a depleted calcium level, in which case my advice would be to use Urticalcin. Nowadays, calcium preparations are often known as silica and much research has been done into the benefits of this mineral. From such research we have learned that not only does silica or a calcium preparation help the circulation, it also lowers the cholesterol level. Again, we have good reason to be thankful to Nature for giving us the means to prevent specific problems that can develop into illnesses such as Raynaud's disease.

A less common illness but one still meriting our attention is lymphoedema. In this condition the build-up of excessive lymph fluid causes swelling in the subcutaneous tissues due to obstruction, or destruction, or hypoplasia, of the lymph vessels. Mostly this causes swelling of the lower legs and especially the ankles. Here again Hyperisan will help and also the remedy Convascillan can be of great benefit in improving the condition of the patient still further. Convascillan's major ingredient is *Convallaria majalis*, or lily of the valley, and is it not wonderful to realise that such an attractive flower gives us the message that it is not poisonous, but if used wisely it will be of service to us. Would you believe, looking at this beautiful spring flower with its deep white colour and fragrant scent among its bright green leaves, that it would make such an excellent natural diuretic? Patients so easily become used to chemical diuretics, which therefore become less effective as time goes on. This natural remedy will effortlessly and harmlessly help to restore the flow of fluids if there are abnormal swellings.

These two remedies stood one particular female patient with lymphoedema in good stead; eventually the treatment was discontinued because she had totally overcome her condition. She told me that her improvement had been such that she had been able to enjoy a swim in the sea again. The salt water of the sea would always be beneficial, in fact the best form of hydrotherapy one could possibly wish for.

This all goes to show that even for difficult conditions we should never give up hope, because even when we think that the end of the road has been reached, Nature may yet have a surprise in store for us.

8

Varicose Veins and Haemorrhoids

SOME TIME AGO I was asked to attend the launch of a new range of herbal remedies. The official event was scheduled to take place in an unexpected haven of peace somewhere in the centre of London. Imagine finding such a horticultural enclave in the centre of one of the busiest cities in the world. The Chelsea Physic Garden is an absolute treat to visit because one comes upon it so totally unexpectedly. It is all the more surprising to find this garden in full bloom when in the background can be heard the drone of the constantly moving traffic. Yet Nature thrives in that garden — and once again I had to admire the innate strength of Nature, which enables it to survive despite the unavoidable atmospherical pollution in that location.

I thoroughly enjoyed the time I was able to spend there. I had been asked to show round a group of journalists and as I did so I told them about some of the wonderful natural remedies that have recently re-emerged after having been neglected for such a long time. I explained the advantages of natural and herbal remedies to the more favoured chemical drugs, which are much more likely to cause undesirable side-effects. On our tour of the garden I pointed out to my listeners an exceptional specimen of a certain tree, called *Ginkgo biloba*. This tree had been badly damaged in the dreadful storms of 1987, during which Kew Gardens had lost so many trees. Obviously, this smaller but no less beautiful garden had not been left unscathed.

This *Ginkgo biloba* tree had been imported into this country about a hundred years ago. Although it had suffered badly in the storms, through careful pruning it had managed to re-establish itself and was indeed one of the most attractive specimens in that garden. The *Ginkgo biloba* tree, commonly known as ginkgo, is the world's oldest living tree species. Although it originates from China, it grows successfully to a ripe old age in many other parts of the world to which it has been transplanted.

Modern scientific analysis has suggested that the reason this species has survived for so long may be that its leaves are packed with highly active chemicals that give the tree unusual resistance to parasites, infections and pollution. The leaves of the ginkgo tree are traditionally harvested in the autumn, just as their colour is changing, and this is exactly the time when they have their highest active concentrations of bioflavonoids. Ginkgo bioflavonoids are now thought to be the most potent of all bioflavonoids and it has been suggested that they have the ability to help maintain the circulation of blood to the brain. Also in advanced cases of varicose veins, *Ginkgo biloba* tablets serve as an especially useful remedy.

Having completed my guided tour that afternoon, despite the throngs of people I found a moment of peace and quiet and listened to the gentle sound of a girl playing the harp and became totally unaware of the background traffic noise. How happy visitors must be to find such peaceful and harmonious surroundings in the centre of such a bustling city!

Such harmony stands the human body and soul in good stead. The body will work very well for us if there is harmony, but such harmony does not appear where it is not wanted or invited. When I worked in China I never failed to be impressed each time I visited Peking by the great temple there, called the Temple of Harmony. So many philosophies of the Chinese are based upon harmony between mind and body. I agree that it is important to find an explanation or a definition for illness or disease, but like the Chinese, I am inclined to believe that all illness or disease is the result of disharmony. The conditions of varicose veins or haemorrhoids are excellent examples of this theory. The blood pushes itself upwards through the veins and where harmony is disturbed the pressure will cause the weaker areas of the veins and arteries to bulge, resulting in varicose veins and haemorrhoids.

Do not make the mistake of writing off varicose veins as an aesthetic flaw because their unsightliness is just one aspect of this condition; it can be an extremely bothersome and painful ailment. Moreover, if these veins bulge significantly, even a minor injury could result in excessive and dangerous bleeding. Neither does the lack of visibility of haemorrhoids make them any easier to bear. I heard from one patient that he had failed an examination because he was suffering from an attack of haemorrhoids during the two days his examination had been scheduled to take place. I can well believe that in such condition you are far from your usual self.

On my tour of the Chelsea Physic Garden I pointed out to my audience as many medicinal herbs as possible. We stopped at the *Hypericum perforatum,* or St John's wort, which just happened to be in full bloom and was carrying a mass of lovely yellow flowers. I then produced a sample of the new herbal range from Heath and Heather that was being launched that day and showed them the small tablets containing the ingredient that had been extracted from the shrub they were admiring even at that moment. The remedy obtained from *Hypericum perforatum* is specifically designed to alleviate circulatory disorders, varicose veins and haemorrhoids.

Some of the journalists expressed amazement and admiration, but I told them that this is not a new science. Heath and Heather is an old and well-established herbal company, as is Napier's of Edinburgh, to name but one more. Dr Vogel has been working with natural and herbal remedies for decades and much of our present knowledge has been handed down by previous generations. Our forebears lived much closer to Nature and they often knew which plants and herbs had medicinal properties.

I also stopped with my group at the *Ruscus aculeatus*, or butcher's broom, which is a beautiful evergreen shrub that originated from the Mediterranean. Only recently we have discovered that the *Ruscus* tincture is capable of clearing congested veins and it is used in the treatment of ulcerated legs and haemorrhoids.

Then I pointed to the horse chestnut tree and told them about the properties of *Aesculus hippocastanum*, which is used in the treatment of circulatory disorders. Generations of people have already used this remedy successfully for exactly such purposes. It makes me wonder how we ever managed to become so side-tracked that we have temporarily disregarded such valuable natural remedies. We should never allow ourselves to forget that God created Nature not only for us to look at with pleasure, but also for us to use to the advantage of our well-being.

People who suffer from haemorrhoids, more commonly known as piles, will know how much of a discomfort this condition can be. It is said that unless we have suffered from haemorrhoids ourselves, we can have little idea of the extent of the suffering they cause. People tend to become especially worried when blood is observed in the stool, and rightly so. Help is certainly needed for this condition. My party had become quite fascinated with the subject by now and I showed them the *Hamamelis virginiana*, or witch hazel, and told them about several of the products that contain witch hazel.

Let us now look back in history, as far back as the Napoleonic Wars. There is a story about Napoleon and his mighty opponent Wellington. Napoleon's power had already started to wane somewhat when, apparently, at one of their meetings on the battlefield Napoleon delayed his attack on Wellington by twenty-four hours. It is understood that Napoleon suffered from haemorrhoids and was in rather a poor state on the day the attack was supposed to have taken place. So that attack was postponed and just look what happened to Europe! No doubt Napoleon suffered a great deal of pain, but for Wellington this was the opportunity to successfully reassemble and engage his troops at Waterloo and break Napoleon's power for ever.

What really is the cause of varicose veins or haemorrhoids? Shop assistants are often warned about the risk of developing varicose veins in the legs as a result of spending long spells on their feet. Yet again, lorry drivers and taxi drivers are more prone to these conditions because they sit in the same position for long periods. Ladies ought to be aware that it is unwise to sit with the legs crossed as this will hinder the circulation of the blood. When the blood from the legs returns to the heart and lungs to gather more oxygen, the weight contracts the muscles and weaker areas in the veins and arteries will come under undue pressure. In the western world both varicose veins and haemorrhoids are much more prevalent than in underdeveloped countries, and if the relevant statistics are to be believed, 20 per cent of the human race suffers from either one or the other of these complaints.

As one gets older the elasticity of the veins is reduced. Also, overweight people carry more fatty tissue and the veins do not receive the required support. Here we have yet another reason to keep down the body weight, especially for people with either a sedentary job or the reverse, when they spend long hours on their feet. This is also one reason why pregnant women have to be very careful, because during pregnancy the enlarged womb will increase the pressure on the veins and this all too often can be the cause of varicose veins or haemorrhoids. Tightly fitted and constrictive clothing, such as corsets, can also be a contributory factor.

Another major cause for concern is constipation. Excess food, and especially excessively spicy food, can be held responsible for haemorrhoids. We have already agreed that even at the best of times this can be a painful and most unpleasant condition, but its symptoms can cause such serious discomfort that a patient may agree to surgery, even though success cannot be guaranteed. Such an operation is nearly always unnecessary. If the correct action is taken in time, the situation can be reversed. Unless there is a really serious prolapse which causes the bowel to be trapped, surgery is usually uncalled for.

Varicose veins, of course, are not restricted to the legs. I have often seen that the testicles can be affected and this can well lead to impotence. Patients with such problems really do need to seek medical advice. Do not suffer in silence out of embarrassment or false shame, because something can be done to help you. Over the years I have treated many sportspeople, and among these were probably more footballers than representatives from other sports. Whenever I have noticed a swelling in the veins, or when the legs appeared to be affected, I have warned them to be careful as even a slight injury could lead to bleeding, a complication that could develop into an infection or ulcers, with possibly disastrous results.

While treating a well-known footballer for a muscular injury, I could not fail to notice that because of the extra muscular movements, the blood flow returning to the heart was coming under severe pressure. Eventually, he was grateful when we managed to sort out his problem. Initially, however, he was not too keen because I had to point out that some of his favourite foods, such as beefburgers and sausages, and sometimes alcohol and nicotine, were definitely not helping his problem, and because he tended to become constipated easily he was heading for a phlebo thrombosis.

I have had to warn many of the older generation about this particular problem, some of whom had already reached the stage that they had experienced a pulmonary embolism. Proper diet and exercise is of the greatest help. We are dealing with the finest material in the human body and a healthy internal lining — *tumeca intima* — and the connective tissues are all necessary to keep the elasticity of the vessels intact.

Statistically, we are led to believe that one in five people in the United Kingdom is troubled by varicose veins and from experience gained at our clinic I can only agree that this problem is definitely on the increase. It would be best if people became aware in the early stages that if they frequently feel a dull ache in the legs, or if they are restless in bed, the circulation is not functioning efficiently. At this early stage the problem can often be easily solved with perhaps some vitamin E or some extra calcium. Prevention is always better than cure and, again, whenever one suspects such problems, please look out for other indications such as cramp during the night, irregular pigmentation of the skin, ulceration, a tender feeling or an oedema. Sometimes these symptoms occur before or during menstruation, but please remain alert to them. Certainly, it is possible to resort to aggressive forms of treatment, such as stripping or injecting the varicose veins, but why not try the natural way first?

I remember one lady who was extremely troubled by haemorrhoids. She was frightened of undergoing an operation because she had been told how very painful the surgery was. I sympathised with her because she was experiencing a great deal of pain and I prescribed an extract of witch hazel, *Hamamelis virginiana*, together with Hyperisan and Urticalcin tablets. This combination, plus witch hazel suppositories, did a wonderful job. I also suggested that she take better care of her diet and advised her accordingly. The main rules here are to avoid pork (including sausages, bacon, ham and gammon), rhubarb, spices, alcohol and chocolates. Reduce the daily intake of coffee and tea; eat plenty of raw and cooked vegetables and, if possible, a salad every day. Include plenty of fibre, fruits, honey, cottage cheese, brown rice and yoghurt. The lady concerned followed these relatively simple guidelines and found that they helped to ease her condition to such an extent that surgery was no longer considered necessary. For both varicose veins and haemorrhoids, it is helpful also to use some water treatments, for example sponging the affected areas with ice-cold water. The external application of a yarrow extract will also soothe the pain caused by haemorrhoids.

Open varicose ulcers must receive immediate attention and great care must be taken in their treatment. My advice would be to use clay poultices daily or to make a poultice from equal amounts of cod liver oil and honey and bandage it in place overnight. I have advised this treatment for many years and it has never disappointed me or the patient. Sometimes it is also helpful to use a fresh comfrey leaf, grated and placed on the affected area, with a clay poultice or a cabbage leaf. For extremely painful conditions mustard flour poultices can be used. Externally, such poultices are often of great benefit and many times my patients have remarked on their excellent results.

I have already written about the role played by nutrition and therefore let us now look at an even more important factor, that is the detoxification of the blood in the bloodstream. So often we discover that certain complaints are due to toxicity in the tissues. We then have to seriously consider following a programme that will normalise the damaged tissue, especially with varicose veins and haemorrhoids problems. In order to detoxify the body one could choose a detoxification programme such as the Rasayana course developed by Dr Vogel.

A relatively new product called Silymarin can also be of great help in a detoxification programme. Milk thistle (*Silybum marianum*, or *Carduus marianus*) is a traditional herbal supplement. Nature's Best has followed up the latest scientific research by formulating a supplement containing the bioflavonoid-rich fruit extract of its most important active ingredient — silymarin. Silymarin can help maintain the health of the liver where an enormous amount of our energy is used. The liver can be thought of as a giant detoxification plant which attempts to filter the toxins and poisons that we introduce — whether accidentally, as in the case of toxins such as pesticides, or intentionally as in the case of alcohol and recreational or prescribed drugs. A number of studies on humans have indicated that the active ingredients of silymarin remain in the liver after oral administration, with only minute amounts being present in the blood circulating round the body.

A sensible fasting programme is an excellent method of detoxification. There are several different ways to fast and the choice depends on personal preference. Some people decide to fast for a few consecutive days, taking only liquids. Others thrive on a programme of fasting for only one day a week. If the latter is chosen it is helpful to be able to stay in bed for the whole day. For breakfast, lunch, dinner and supper take a glass of juice. If it is not possible to spend the day in bed, at least try to take it easy. The same regime should be followed one day every week.

In China I have heard very good reports on an interesting method of detoxification based on a theory that was first published in an article written by a Japanese professor some years ago.

Drinking six large tumblers of water at one time renders the colon more effective in forming more new and fresh blood. As a result of insufficient exercise of the colonic tract, man feels exhausted and becomes sick. The colon, or large intestine, of an adult can be eight feet long and is capable of absorbing the nutrients taken several times a day. If the colon is clean, then the nutrients will be completely absorbed by the meucosa folds, which will turn them into fresh blood. This blood is responsible for curing our ailments and is considered as a prime power in the improvement of our health. In other words the "Water Therapy" will make us healthy and prolong our mortal lives.

A sick person might find it difficult to drink large quantities of water, but should persevere. Wherever possible, try to take exercise after drinking the water. Bedridden people who are unable to get up and do some exercises after drinking the water should practise deep inspiration and expiration while lying in bed and massage their stomachs with the aim of making the water inside the colon flow so as to wash and clean the meucosa folds. Some people will experience loose bowels and may have to urinate maybe as much as three times in one hour. However, after three or four days, the trouble will be eliminated.

After the course some herbal teas or specific herbal tablets may be used and many patients have managed to bring their problems under control with this method. In the case of varicose veins and/or haemorrhoids it would also be advisable to take a vitamin supplement and I would suggest 500–1,000 mg of vitamin C daily and up to 600 IU of vitamin E. This will help to reduce the swelling and pain and prevent phlebitis.

It is most interesting to see what Nature has to offer, thinking back to that little walk in the Chelsea Physic Garden right in the heart of London. Do we ever stop to consider if the price today's society is paying for its convenience and comfort is too extravagant in terms of health problems? Yet Nature still offers us a helping hand. Let us try to keep diet and stress under control and the price may yet come down!

9

Blood Pressure

SO FAR, WE have looked at the cardiovascular system and various related problems and I have tried to give some simple explanations of these. Now let us move on to the subject of blood pressure and its relation to some of these problems. On this topic I have explained how the heart and lungs, by way of the veinous system, receive blood for cleansing and recharging. The blood is pumped through the lungs where it will be detoxified and at the same time regains fresh oxygen. If this process is in harmony then there is a degree of flexibility and elasticity. The effectiveness of this process, then, completely depends on how much pressure there is on the arteries and how freely the blood can flow.

Blood pressure is measured with a sphygmomanometer and is always expressed in two values, that is the systolic pressure, which is the pressure in the arteries after the beat, and the pause between the beats when the inter-arterial pressure is taken, called the diastolic pressure. One can actually liken the body's system for controlling the blood pressure to the central heating system of a house. With a heating system we see that the electric pump forces the water through the radiators. The main pipe leaving the pump leads to a number of smaller pipes and the pressure from the pump determines the amount of water sent on its journey through the house. The size of the pipes controls the amount of water passing through, while a change of pressure obviously allows more or less water to flow through the pipes. Corrosion or dirt are two factors that can bring a change in the pressure; in other words the pressure indicates whether or not the system is in good working order and if the pipes or blood vessels become clogged, the mobility of the water or blood will be impaired. If this is the case, the efficiency, whether of the heating system or of the circulation in the human body, is greatly decreased.

It only requires a simple act to measure the blood pressure and we obtain a clear impression from this of how healthy the blood circulation is and how well the heart is coping. This is dependent on the viscosity, or thickness, of the blood and this factor should never be underestimated. Blood pressure varies from one person to another and it is difficult to say exactly which reading is acceptable and which is not. In addition, blood pressure is rarely consistent and can change from one minute to the next. On average, at the age of twenty-one, a blood pressure reading can safely vary from about 105 over 62 to 140 over 82. Therefore a younger person whose reading is higher than 140 over 82 is quite likely to be heading for problems and would be wise to take action as soon as possible.

How relevant is what we eat and drink to high blood pressure? This question reminds me of a young man in his early twenties, recently married and with a responsible job. When he came to me he had not felt well enough to go to work for quite some time. I took his blood pressure and the reading was so high that I became anxious to see him leave the consulting room alive. When we discussed his diet I was so shocked that I asked to speak to his wife. I asked her if she loved him and she looked strangely at me before assuring me that of course she did. I told her that if she wanted to keep her husband she would be wise to help him change his diet. When he first came to see me he weighed in excess of sixteen stones, but between the three of us we have now managed to bring his weight down to a healthy level. He has also stopped the habit of taking self-prescribed drugs. He admitted he only ever took these to make him feel better, but feels no need for them now that he is fit and healthy again and has returned to work. Occasionally I see him at the weekend when he is out on his bike; this is his way of solving his previous lack of exercise.

The above case confirms that diet has a definite bearing on one's health, especially when you consider that this young man was in the habit of eating a fried breakfast of bacon and eggs every morning and admitted to being liberal with the condiments, especially salt. His breakfast certainly contained all the ingredients to raise one's blood pressure. Remember, blood pressure is vital to health and life. High blood pressure can become a real threat to life, as indeed can low blood pressure, and the balance between the systolic and diastolic pressure determines the expectancy of life.

There are, of course, many reasons why the blood pressure may rise. These can be dietary as explained above, or related to stress, degeneration or old age, but also it can have a strong link with one's emotions or pressures of life. In the Far East, where people tend to take life easier, I have come across very few patients with high blood pressure. Especially when I ask people to list their symptoms, it always amazes me to see the difference, because so often in the West those symptoms would include one or more of the following: tingling sensations, buzzing in the ears, dizziness, headaches, irritability, aggression, tiredness, tingling sensitivity around the mouth or nose bleeds, all of which indicate the likelihood of raised blood pressure. Please consult a medical practitioner if you recognise several of these symptoms.

A middle-aged lady once consulted me about a non-related matter. I asked her when she last had her blood pressure taken and she informed me that she had no problem with her blood pressure so there was little need to have that checked. I looked at her and asked her to allow me to look at the swellings, or oedema, on her legs and whether she considered that her face was swollen. She admitted that she looked somewhat puffy and when I was allowed to take her blood pressure, the reading was indeed extremely high. Such a build-up of fluid that causes swellings on the legs can be serious and if this is due to a kidney problem, one has to be especially careful.

I asked her why she was so adamant about not having her blood pressure taken and once again I recognised the fear I sometimes come across in patients. Very often this is an indication that they know that something is wrong, but by not admitting it or not having it confirmed, they try to avoid facing reality. In tears, she told me that she had been under a great deal of stress because of an unhappy relationship and she had also noticed that recently she had become more aggressive and angry. She also admitted to bouts of anxiety. Often if there is a tendency towards poor eating habits, these are the times at which the person concerned will particularly crave those food items that lie at the root of the problem. When that craving has been temporarily satisfied, the patient will be happy for a short period, only to find that the same situation recurs again and again. I often recognise this pattern in patients with high blood pressure, who usually appear to be more or less addicted to salt. I always try to explain to them that excess salt will cause their pulse rate to rise, which is tantamount to inviting problems. Apart from everything else, the kidneys have a great aversion to salt, as it places them under great strain to process it.

Once again I must say that when I worked in China I saw only very few cases of high blood pressure. It is reckoned that unpolished brown rice, a major constituent of their diet, is of the greatest natural regulators of blood pressure. In fact, the Chinese claim that it is *the* most important aid. They claim, to my mind quite justifiably, that unpolished rice is the best yin and yang food possible as it helps to restore the elasticity in the arteries and enhances the circulation. However, in order to be effective in this way unpolished rice must be cooked correctly. To this end I have included a suitable recipe below.

Place the desired quantity of rice in a casserole or Pyrex dish. Pour over some milk or, preferably, water. Having preheated the oven to the highest temperature, place the dish of rice in the oven and leave for only 10–15 minutes at this temperature. Then switch off the oven and leave the rice inside for 5–6 hours. Chop some vegetables, such as parsley, chicory, celery and cress, and mix these through the rice with a little garlic salt or soya sauce. When required, heat the rice through again. I can only say that when prepared in this way, unpolished rice is possibly better for our health than any other nutrient.

People who are susceptible to high blood pressure should try to exclude the following food items, or at least keep their use to a minimum: salt, sugar, spices, alcohol, chocolate, pork in any shape or form, butter, cream and fats. The more natural the diet the quicker there will be a response, that is a lowering of the blood pressure, and one will start to feel better. Kitchen herbs, too, can be extremely helpful and it is wonderful how beneficial such everyday ingredients can be. On the front cover of this book is featured an illustration of the *Allium ursinum*, or wild leek, and a patient with high blood pressure will never be disappointed when using this.

It never ceases to amaze me that this strong and at the same time pleasant-smelling plant is so beneficial in regulating the blood pressure and that is the reason I decided to choose it to illustrate the cover of this book.

The use of buckwheat is also becoming more widespread and this too has given great relief in cases of high blood pressure. Together with onion, garlic and marjoram it will help to balance the blood pressure. For the heart we can use the hawthorn berry — *Crataegus oxyacantha*. Dr Vogel has used this as the main ingredient in his remedy called Crataegisan and this remedy is not only helpful in the treatment of angina pectoris, but also of high blood pressure.

This reminds me of an elderly lady from Ireland who had travelled across on the ferry to see me. In a corner of her bag she had neatly tucked away a little pouch containing some berries. She carefully opened this small pouch and showed me the contents. She told me that her mother used to use these berries for high blood pressure and heart complaints and she wanted to ask me whether it was safe for her to use them. The berries she showed me were hawthorn berries, but she had not dared to take them without first obtaining professional confirmation. On looking her over I immediately decided to check her blood pressure and when I did so, I found it to be very high indeed. I had to prescribe some much stronger remedies in order to try and bring down her blood pressure as quickly as possible. She admitted that her doctor had prescribed remedies for her but she was allergic to them and now her doctor had more or less given up on her. I asked her about her daily habits and learned that she was one of those people who love baking and always had a supply of biscuits and cakes at hand for visitors and then joined them in this feast with her cup of tea. She believed in eating good solid meals and it was easy to see how she had caused so many problems for herself.

I prescribed some natural remedies and she was very willing to take my advice on dietary matters. She promised to reduce her intake of fats and salt and I also explained that especially when one gets older it is advisable to reduce the intake of animal protein and that this in itself would benefit the blood.

Dr Vogel often used the allegoric story of the fire. Nutrients are to the body what fuel is to a fire. Coal burns brightly on the fire and leaves ashes and cinders, while wood leaves only dust. Carbohydrates can be compared to wood logs; they supply the body with nutrients and the waste matter is disposed of in the normal manner through the excretory organs. Animal protein, however, is comparable to coal, which leaves crystals, cinders and stones. Impurities left in the fire can be equated to the crystals and fats that are left behind in our system to affect the blood pressure or lead to a hardening of the arteries.

The little Irish lady was very happy when I told her on her following visit that she could safely take a few of those little berries each day. She still writes occasionally to reassure me that she is keeping well and how happy she is to follow the simple advice I gave her.

If the blood pressure is very high it might be helpful to take some Arterioforce, as mentioned earlier, and some *Viscum album*, or extract from the mistletoe. I could fill a book on the beneficial properties of mistletoe and I have indeed sung its praises in my book *Traditional Home and Herbal Remedies*. It has been known for centuries that mistletoe is a wonderful remedy for many ailments, including high blood pressure. Physicians like Hippocrates and Dioscorides found mistletoe a valuable remedial plant. The Druids called it "the plant that heals all ills", which may be a slight exaggeration, but it has proved to be extremely useful in the treatment of high blood pressure. Dr Vogel's Viscasan, which consists mostly of *Viscum album*, has indeed given tremendous assistance in such cases.

High blood pressure is often considered as an indicator of disease, especially when there is concern about the arteries. If in doubt, do ask your practitioner for a test, which will soon show up any other conditions that may lie at the root of the blood pressure problem. So often I have to come to the conclusion that high blood pressure is self-inflicted, because if we allow stress to take hold of us and we do not try to put a stop to it, then we can only expect to suffer its effects. Of course, reducing stress is easier said than done, but if we positively set our mind to it we may decide to practise some relaxation exercises or even undergo counselling. Always remember that no one else can do it for us. The next blood pressure test will soon confirm that we are on the right road.

Take some time right now to consider if you really need so many refined food products. Do you need all that excess sugar? Is your alcohol intake really as low as you would make yourself believe? Do you drink too much coffee, tea or chocolate? Do you really eat your meals at regular times? Is it necessary to spend so much time watching television? Does your diet contain too many animal products? There is nothing to be lost by asking yourself these questions and when you answer them truthfully you will soon know if there is room for improvement.

When a change in diet is required, it is often easier to follow dietary guidelines for a fixed period, after which time you can gradually introduce touches of your own. This will give you the initial stimulation that is so often appreciated. The diet below is directed towards a vegetarian regime, but as I have said, this can be adapted in time to suit your individual requirements.

Diet for regulating the blood pressure
General notes
Do not exceed the weekly allowance of:
—4 oz Outline margarine or low fat spread
—3 eggs

Do not exceed the daily allowance of:
—1/2 pint of Marvel or skimmed milk
For coffee and tea use part of the daily milk allowance.
Lunch should be accompanied by a green salad.
Dinner should include a medium helping of vegetables of your choice.

Day 1

Breakfast:
One shredded wheat, 1/4 pint Marvel or skimmed milk, 1 oz bread, one apple

Lunch:
Small glass of vegetable juice, 1 oz bread, one egg (scrambled), 1/4 pint Marvel or skimmed milk, one orange

Dinner:
3 oz potatoes, half a tin of Cadbury's Soya choice casserole, one banana

Day 2

Breakfast:
Half a grapefruit, 1 oz muesli, 1/4 pint Marvel or skimmed milk, 1 oz bread

Lunch:
Small glass of tomato juice, 1 oz bread, 4 oz cottage cheese, 1/4 pint Marvel or skimmed milk

Dinner: 3 oz potatoes, 3 oz Granose Soyapro Weiners, one tub of natural low fat yoghurt

Day 3

Breakfast:
Half a grapefruit, 1 oz (dry) porridge, 1/4 pint Marvel or skimmed milk, 1 oz bread

Lunch:
Small glass of tomato juice, macaroni cheese made with 1/2 oz dry macaroni and 1 oz Cheddar cheese, 1/4 pint Marvel or skimmed milk, one orange

Dinner:
Three tablespoons cooked rice, 6 oz Mapleton's rissoles in tomatoes, one tub of natural low fat yoghurt, one apple

Day 4

Breakfast:
One Weetabix, 1/4 pint Marvel or skimmed milk, 1 oz bread, one banana

Lunch:
Home-made clear vegetable soup, 1 oz bread spread generously with honey, 1/4 pint Marvel or skimmed milk, one orange

Dinner:
Three tablespoons sweetcorn, 3 oz Granose Soyapro chicken, one apple, one tub of natural low fat yoghurt

Day 5

Breakfast:
One orange, 1 oz Fru-grains, 1 oz bread, 1/4 pint Marvel or skimmed milk

Lunch:
Marmite drink (one teaspoon), 1 oz bread, 1 oz Cheddar cheese, 1/4 pint Marvel or skimmed milk, one apple

Dinner:
Three tablespoons boiled rice, half a tin of Appleford's meatless goulash, one banana, one tub of natural low fat yoghurt

Day 6

Breakfast:
1 oz All Bran, 1/4 pint Marvel or skimmed milk, 1 oz bread, one orange

Lunch:
Small glass of vegetable juice, 1 oz bread, two poached eggs, half a grapefruit

Dinner:
Home-made clear vegetable soup, three tablespoons boiled rice, 7 oz can of Appleford's meatless curry, one tub of natural low fat yoghurt, one orange

Day 7

Breakfast:
Half a grapefruit, 1 oz cornflakes, 1/4 pint Marvel or skimmed milk, 1 oz bread

Lunch:
Small glass of vegetable juice, 1 oz bread, 1 oz Edam cheese, 1/4 pint Marvel or skimmed milk, one banana

Dinner:
Three tablespoons sweetcorn, 2 oz nut rissoles, one tub of natural low fat yoghurt, half a grapefruit

Very often, high blood pressure is related to the weight of the person concerned and in many cases a sincere attempt at following a weight-reduction diet will help to reduce the blood pressure. The following dietary guidelines are designed as an advisory tool and allow room for individual choice. With some careful consideration they can be adapted so that the whole family can still sit around the table and eat the same meals.

Suggested day's menu for the family
Daily allowances (per person)
Milk (fresh) — 1/2 pint or 1 pint of Marvel
Wholewheat bread — 3 oz
Meat — 4 oz, or fish — 6 oz
Fruit — three portions

Weekly allowances (per person)
Butter — 1/4 lb or margarine
Cheese — 1/2 lb

Exchanges for 1 oz bread
Potato — one medium
Crispbread, crackers, water biscuits — two
Breakfast cereal — 1 oz of any sort except sugar-coated
Cooked rice — two dessertspoons
Plain biscuits or oatcakes — two

Breakfast:
Grapefruit or unsweetened fruit juice
Egg (poached, boiled, scrambled, omelette)
1 oz wholewheat bread or toast, plus butter from weekly allowance

Mid-morning:
Tea or coffee

Lunch:
Lean meat, fish, egg, cheese

Vegetable or salad
1 oz wholewheat bread (or exchange), plus butter from weekly allowance
Fresh fruit — one portion
Tea or coffee

Mid-afternoon:
Tea or coffee

Dinner:
Clear vegetable soup or tomato juice
Lean meat, fish, egg, cheese
Vegetable or salad
1 oz wholewheat bread (or exchange), plus butter from weekly allowance
Fresh fruit — one portion
Tea or coffee

Bedtime:
Tea or coffee

Foods to be avoided or limited
Sugar and its products:
Glucose, sweets, chocolate, ice-cream, sweetened yoghurt, jam, marmalade, lemon curd, treacle, syrup, puddings, lemonade, squashes, proprietary milk drinks, tinned fruits

White flour and its products:
Cakes, sweet biscuits, pastries, crumpets, doughnuts, scones, buns, dumplings, pies, bridies, sausage rolls, spaghetti, macaroni, thick gravies and sauces, thick pickles and chutneys, tinned and packet soups, thick soups

Fatty foods:
Dripping, lard, oil, salad cream, cream, fatty meat, sausages, fried foods, black pudding, fishcakes, fish fingers, rissoles, chips, roast potatoes, potato crisps

Miscellaneous items:
Honey, nuts, alcohol, evaporated or condensed milk, Sorbitol, slimming biscuits, diabetic foods and squashes, processed meat

Variety is the spice of life
Meats (4 oz daily, cooked any way except fried):
Beef, chicken, corned beef, duck, kidney, lamb, liver, mutton, rabbit, sweetbreads, tongue, tripe, turkey, veal

Fish (6 oz daily, cooked any way except fried):
Cod, crab, haddock, halibut, hake, herring, kippers, lobster, ling, mackerel, mussels, oysters, pilchards, prawns, salmon, sardines, shrimps, trout, tuna

Eggs (1 daily):
Poached, boiled, scrambled, omelette

Cheese (1 oz daily):
Caerphilly, Camembert, Cheddar, Cheshire, cottage cheese (4 oz), Danish Blue, Edam, Gruyere, Leicester, Parmesan, Roquefort, Stilton, Wensleydale, Smoked Austrian

Vegetables:
(Unlimited)
Artichokes, asparagus, aubergines, bean sprouts, Brussels sprouts, beetroot, broccoli, cabbage (red, savoy, spring, winter), carrots, cauliflower, celery, chicory, courgettes, cress, cucumber, lettuce, marrow, mushrooms, onions, parsley, parsnip, red and green peppers, pickles (beetroot, dill, gherkins, red cabbage), pimentoes, French and runner beans, radishes, spinach, spring onions, swede, tomatoes

(In moderation)
Peas, beans (baked, butter, broad, haricot), sweetcorn

Fruit (3 portions daily):

Apple	— average	Peach	— average
Apricots	— 2 fresh	Pear	— average
Avocado	— half	Pineapple	— 1 slice, fresh
Banana	— small	Plums	— 2
Blackberries	— 4 oz	P'granate	— average
Cooking apple	— large	Prunes	— 6 stewed
(baked or stewed)		Raisins	— 1 oz
Cherries	— 4 oz	Raspberries	— 4 oz
Dates	— 1 oz	Rhubarb	— 4 oz
Damsons	— 10	Strawberries	— 4 oz
Gooseberries	— 10	Sultanas	— 1 oz
Grapefruit	— 1/2 large	Tangerines	— 2
Grapes	— 3 oz	Orange	— average
Melon	— 1 slice	Unsweetened	— 4 oz
		fruit juice	

Drinks:
Tea, Russian tea, herb tea, coffee, Bovril, Oxo, Marmite, soda water, PLJ, tomato juice, water, Energen, 1 Cal., Slimline drinks, low-calorie tonic

Seasonings:
Salt, pepper, vinegar, mustard, lemon juice, herbs, spices, Worcestershire sauce

In addition to diet, it is also sensible to think about how much exercise you take. Do some more walking and practise breathing exercises while out in the fresh air, so that you can inhale deeply and receive your full quota of oxygen. This is extremely important if you are prone to irregular blood pressure readings.

It is also important to look at your intake of vitamins, minerals and trace elements. Some of the vitamins will help to regulate high blood pressure and it has also recently become known that a low level of choline in the body can cause the blood pressure to rise. Choline is found in fish, soya beans, yeast, nuts, liver and wheatgerm, and extra quantities of this component can also be taken in the form of lecithin. In some cases of high blood pressure it has been established that the choline level was relatively low and if this is the case measures can be taken to counteract this through the diet.

High blood pressure should never be ignored, but neither should low blood pressure. In its own way low blood pressure can cause anxiety and excessive tiredness and this also needs to be attended to. Very often I have seen that the old biblical plant hyssop has been of great help here, possibly combined with some extra vitamin E. Hyssop tablets are available in the Bioforce range of natural remedies and these are highly recommended for treating loss or lack of energy, fatigue, a general feeling of tiredness and listlessness. It seems, however, that they are especially effective as a preventative remedy for low blood pressure.

Hypertension and hypotension, that is high blood pressure and low blood pressure, have one thing in common: they affect the function of the blood — the symbol of life. So, let us take care to restore the correct balance.

I notice among my patients that people with low blood pressure are subject to anaemia, a condition I will consider in greater detail in the next chapter.

10

Anaemia

ANAEMIA IS A WORD that is often used when people appear pale or listless, but do we really know what anaemia is all about? To put it simply, anaemia is a condition in which there is a reduction of the number of red blood corpuscles and/or of haemoglobin in the blood. The result of this is to diminish the blood's capacity to transport oxygen. The cause of anaemia may be an inadequate production of red cells, but it can also be caused by an excessive loss of blood.

Pernicious anaemia is a specific form of anaemia characterised by lesions of the spinal cord, weakness, a sore tongue, numbness in the arms and legs, and diarrhoea, and this is considered to be associated with inadequate absorption of vitamin B_{12}. Unless a diagnosis of pernicious anaemia has been confirmed, there are many ways that anaemia can be helped. But let us first look at why it should occur and the reason behind it.

Blood is a liquid compound of blood plasma containing red blood cells, white blood cells and platelets.

This liquid takes care of the vital transport and efficient distribution of nutrients and oxygen to all parts of the body. Blood circulates through the heart, arteries, veins and capillaries, depending firstly on the red blood cells, called the erythrocytes, which contain the haemoglobin and carry oxygen, giving the blood its familiar red colour, and secondly the white blood cells, also called leukocytes (see also page 77).

We should be grateful to the blood because this red liquid is essential for the nourishment of tissues and cells, while in addition it carries anti-toxins and other ingredients which help to ward off invaders.

A normal adult has approximately 8–10 pints of blood and it is, of course, of great importance that the amount of blood is kept to the required level and is of such a quality that it can fulfil all the functions it is supposed to do. If we look at what is required of the blood, it is no wonder that it is often called the "elixir of life". We ourselves are responsible for keeping the quality of the blood up to standard and wherever possible for improving it and certainly encouraging it in its task with some of the remedies Nature has to offer.

I remember a young lady who became very fond of soup made with stinging nettles. She had once been told that this plant was a sensible supplement and for those of you who have never tried it, I can assure you that it is completely edible. Cheese with nettles also tastes good and it is certainly worth giving it a try. What this young lady did not know was that by eating nettles she had improved the quality of her blood and although once she had been slightly anaemic, the increased level of haemoglobin had actually cured her anaemia.

Slight deficiencies of certain nutrients could result in a drastic breakdown of the haemoglobin and a reduction of physical stamina. This has happened in some parts of the world as a result of vitamin E deficiency and can also easily happen when insufficient fresh vegetables are eaten, such as spinach, endive, lettuce, alfalfa or cress. This is also the reason why Herbamare salt is better for us than normal salt, because Herbamare salt contains valuable supplementary nutrients. Its use will indeed help to maintain the correct level of haemoglobin.

Herbamare is a herbal seasoning salt from the Bioforce range and is especially nutritious as it contains fresh, organically grown herbs and unrefined sea salt plus natural iodine obtained from kelp. It is made according to the original formula of the famous Swiss naturopath Dr A. Vogel. The fresh herbs are combined with natural sea salt and allowed to "steep" for 6–8 weeks before the moisture is removed by a special vacuum process at a low temperature. This slow, careful process allows all the good qualities, the aroma and taste to be absorbed by the sea salt. Use Herbamare at the table, in cooking or any time you want the taste and aroma of fresh herbs. The ingredients of Herbamare are sea salt, celery leaves, leeks, celery root, cress (water and garden), onions, chives, parsley, lovage, basil, marjoram, rosemary, thyme and kelp.

An anaemic condition can also develop as a result of an iron deficiency, when fresh vegetables containing iron are not used regularly enough. Anaemia in itself is not an illness, but it is a condition that deserves our attention to avoid it becoming a symptom of an illness.

One young person looked sceptically at me when, after having pulled her eyelid down and having looked at her tongue and the colour of her skin, I told her that she could well be anaemic. She bluntly asked me how I could tell without having done a proper blood test. Of course, that is a reasonable question, but the body gives us signals that anaemic conditions could be gaining a foothold. She asked for an explanation and I told her that red blood cells remain in the bloodstream for roughly four months before being used by the liver and the spleen. If too many of the red blood cells are degraded, then the patient's blood will not be able to transport sufficient oxygen; the heart will then be required to beat faster and anaemia will set in. An external indication that can easily be detected is to pull back the lower eyelid and if this is very pale, the person concerned is most likely anaemic.

Approximately 15 per cent of the blood is made up of haemoglobin, although in males this percentage is slightly higher than in females. I told this girl that a blood test would doubtless confirm my diagnosis and I felt that she should take action immediately. She admitted to experiencing a persistent weariness and that, mentally as well physically, everything seemed to require effort. I explained that the brain is highly sensitive to anaemic tendencies and not to be surprised if she occasionally fainted. She told me that she had noticed that when she did any physical exercise or if she had to concentrate very hard, her heart started to beat faster and she also felt nauseous. These are classic symptoms of anaemia and the subsequent tests indeed confirmed that this young girl was considerably anaemic. When I investigated her case further it became clear that she had a deficient dietary regime and certainly lacked sufficient iron and vitamin B_{12}. In olden days it would often be recommended to eat raw liver or other iron-rich products to overcome such problems. A very good remedy to use in these circumstances to help the role of the red blood cells is folic acid and, for some reason or another, I have found that in Scotland many people have a low level of folic acid, which could partly explain why I have so many rheumatic and arthritic patients under treatment.

If our blood is healthy we can afford to lose a fair amount of it because it is capable of quickly replenishing itself, but when there is a problem this becomes usually somewhat more difficult. In any case of bleeding the bone marrow quickly makes up the losses and the body takes it upon itself to correct the matter, but especially with younger women who experience excessive blood loss through menstruation, I often recommend an iron supplement. I have found that Vital Iron Plus from Nature's Best is generally well tolerated and effective. This is an iron food supplement with three important co-factors formulated to combine harmoniously with other nutrients. The Vital Iron Plus formula contains vitamin C, iron, vitamin B₁₂ and folic acid.

I would quite happily say that blood must be considered to be one of the most costly liquids and therefore deserves every care and attention. Blood must not only be regarded as a liquid that enables our body to function; it is worth remembering that without blood there will be no life. Let us have a look at the dietary ingredients we have at our disposal to help the blood to do its function properly.

In many parts of the world kohlrabi leaves have proved to be very helpful as have spinach, endive and various other fresh green vegetables. The very best stimulant I know must be beetroot. Numerous health problems have been solved with beetroot juice and it is invaluable for improving the quality of blood. Oddly enough, the beetroot belongs to the spinach family and it has superb properties which not only improve the condition of the blood, but also benefit the digestion. Moreover, beetroot also has natural antibiotic properties. Please note that beetroot should always be eaten raw. It breaks my heart when I see how beetroot is steeped in vinegar to conserve it, because to me this is an abuse of the medicinal properties of this marvellous vegetable, as its beneficial characteristics are destroyed by this process. Beetroot has high contents of copper, iron, silicone and, when mixed with onion, the highest silicic acid content of the vitamin B complex. It also contains betamine — a nitrogen donator activator and stimulator of the phosphate synthesis of choline — and it encourages the detoxification of the blood and the build-up of haemoglobin.

Bearing in mind the above information, we will understand that the blood needs to receive certain ingredients and these are mostly obtained from a nutritional diet. In this context, some extra carrot juice, beetroot juice or other vegetable juices are highly recommended. Especially for patients who are in need of a surgical operation, and who refuse to accept blood transfusions for whichever reason, apart from some glucose a very good remedy is to take four dried pears two or three times a week. Soak the pears overnight in red wine or red grape juice and eat them as a dessert. Not only is this a healthy practice but also a very tasty one. Other good ways to improve the quality of the blood include drinking pure grape juice, with a raw egg beaten in it, or taking alfalfa tablets.

One of the best remedies must be Galeopsis, which is available from Bioforce. This is a fresh herb preparation which has an expectorant effect in cases of bronchial cough, problems with the respiratory tract and asthma. This remedy's major ingredient is *Galeopsis ochroleuca*, or the hemp nettle. This, too, will be of tremendous help in building up the haemoglobin, especially when it is taken in combination with wheatgerm capsules.

The older generation will probably remember elderberry wine, although perhaps with mixed feelings. Some of you will have enjoyed it as a beverage, while for others it may have been taken as a medical tonic. It was claimed that elderberry wine cleansed the blood and cleared it of impurities. There was indeed great wisdom in this because the elderberry does have great cleansing properties. This fact was already widely known among the Greeks and Romans and therefore a number of their traditional and religious rituals paid tribute to the elderberry. The elderberry is still greatly appreciated for its cleansing capabilities in alternative medicine and is also successfully used to achieve extra weight loss. The elderberry has provided us with a very useful remedy for the digestion and the blood circulation. Cleansing and detoxification enable the blood to perform its mysterious job.

It is also of great importance, when dealing with anaemia problems, to consider the possibility of a ribo-flavin deficiency, usually caused by a reduced activation of folic acid. This can be prevented by taking about 10 mg of vitamin B_2 daily. For iron deficiency, take at least 100 mg of vitamin C in combination with each dose of iron supplement. For haemolytic anaemia conditions, caused by vitamin E deficiency, take approximately 200–300 IU daily in water-soluble form, although adults can take up to 600 IU. Megablastic anaemia also needs folic acid. Pernicious anaemia responds well to vitamin B_{12}, but because of its malabsorption it will have to be injected. Pyridoxine deficiency can sometimes be caused by taking the contra-ceptive pill and this condition can be prevented by taking 25 mg of vitamin B_6 daily. Sickle cell anaemia usually responds well to 400–600 IU of vitamin E daily. The so-called Mediterranean anaemia can mostly be cleared by taking up to 600 IU of vitamin E daily.

Most people will have heard about royal jelly because it has been receiving a substantial amount of publicity lately. In many cases royal jelly will also be beneficial to the anaemic patient. This is an excellent dietary supplement and is a natural substance with properties that cannot be introduced scientifically. Because royal jelly contains vitamin B, it will always help the anaemic patient and they are often advised to take 150–200 mg daily. Several tests have proved that the haemoglobin will also increase with the use of royal jelly.

This vital mysterious red liquid — the blood — that pulses through our veins to keep us alive, deserves all the care and nourishment we can lavish on it and it will repay our efforts with worthwhile energy.

11

Prevention

IT IS A WELL-KNOWN fact in medicine that even minor symptoms can lead to drastic conditions, which perhaps may not be fully understood until many years later. The same goes for medical knowledge and acceptance, although it would be narrow minded to limit this generalisation to medical knowledge. Innovative ideas or principles, in many fields, are often scoffed at until a wider acceptance has been gained, when suddenly it becomes obvious and is heralded as the discovery of the decade or the century.

If I had to name one single thing that has amazed me in all the years I have been practising medicine it must be the emergence and acceptance of the beneficial properties of the seeds of the evening primrose. Not long ago I learned from several of the manufacturers who use oil of evening primrose in their remedies that I was actually the first practitioner in the United Kingdom to work with the evening primrose. I can remember that when I came to this country some twenty years ago there appeared to be no knowledge of the fantastic properties and characteristics of the very small seeds of this plant. However, my grandmother often advised the use of its seeds, so she must have known. Poets have written about the vital powers of the evening primrose, but that the seeds in modern times would become so valuable in the treatment of deficiencies, no one could ever have predicted.

I happily prescribed oil of evening primrose during my early years in Scotland, even though I was often maligned for it. Quite a few times I was told that doing so smelled of "quackery". I remember one occasion when a doctor asked me what in the world I thought I was playing at and who did I think I could fool. I maintain that the sceptical attitude did not really bother me because I was certain that evening primrose worked and I continued to prescribe this remedy. My patients' reports of their improvement were all the proof I might have needed and, indeed, eventually this remedy has become widely accepted.

Let me tell you about the lady who had already undergone several surgical operations and who was once again hospitalised. The surgeon who had performed the previous operations remarked on the speed of her recovery and how good her blood circulation was. She gave credit for this to the fact that she had used oil of evening primrose capsules and this aroused his interest. He was so impressed with her condition that he decided to find out more about this remedy. When he decided that this remedy was worth further investigation he wrote an article about it and this was the beginning of the recognition of the medical value of oil of evening primrose. Gradually, an increasing number of alternative practitioners started to work with it and more research was undertaken. On my travels I am often heralded as the "pioneer of the evening primrose", whose claims have come true. I am not unhappy about this, but neither do I forget the times when I had been scorned.

I remember receiving a telephone call from a hospital specialist who actually burst into laughter when I told him that I used oil of evening primrose for menopausal complaints, as well as for circulatory problems, hormonal imbalance, skin problems, asthmatic complaints and generally as a preventative measure. He accused me of having found a panacea.

Not so long ago, I learned to my pleasure that at that same hospital where this specialist is employed, oil of evening primrose capsules are now frequently prescribed and, to make a long story short, when recently I read about claims that oil of evening primrose may be beneficial to people fighting alcohol addiction, I could not help smiling. Oil of evening primrose capsules are now available on the National Health and are widely prescribed by general practitioners. My years of battling against disbelief and ridicule have not been for nothing. My belief in the vital power of Nature has not been in vain. I am happy with the eventual outcome and although I would not think of claiming any honour for this myself, I am often told how appreciated my efforts are in helping to get this product established in Britain. It makes one appreciate how right the Scottish poet Robert Burns was when he wrote to Dr Moore that the blunders and mistakes we have made are mainly through our ignorance. Because we did not know and were ignorant about this remedy, we immediately refuted the possibility of its benefits. The other day I listened to an interview with a famous medical personality who was asked for his opinion on homoeopathy and he answered that it was not effective. In reply to the question as to whether he had ever worked with it, he had to admit that this was not the case. It remains a mystery to me how we can possibly judge something that we have not tried ourselves. I often encounter the same attitude during my lectures to hospital students and staff — and usually the criticism comes from the ones who have never tried it and have never bothered to investigate it either.

However, we have reason to be grateful that at last the vital power of the evening primrose has been acknowledged. These little seeds contain powerful properties that can change the course of some extremely persistent illnesses or health problems.

Why do I embellish on this aspect yet again? Simply because this chapter is dedicated to the many ways in which we can prevent heart and blood circulatory problems. Prevention is still better than cure, so why not, once in a while, take a course of this marvellous and harmless remedy.

Remember that the recognition of the usefulness of digitalis was coincidental, just as many other now acceptable remedies were discovered accidentally. What has only recently become known is that the evening primrose seeds contain an extremely rare ingredient called gamma linoleic acid (GLA). Nowadays this is considered a particularly valuable asset because in our present environment we are very much in need of it. Gamma linoleic acid is converted in the body to a physiological substance called prostaglandin, or PGE1, and this has a highly effective action. We find GLA in other products and this is one of the reasons that people with cholesterol problems are so often advised to include oats in their diet, because oats also contain some GLA, as do certain kinds of berries, for example, blackcurrant and borage. The evening primrose is one of the richest sources of GLA, however, and although this particular information was not always known to us, we do know that the evening primrose always serves to boost our health.

From the various notes I have been left by my relatives I learned that they considered it a drawback that no research had been done into the medical properties of the evening primrose. In recent years this has been rectified and research is still going on. I am certainly not planning to devote this whole chapter to the evening primrose and will also look at various other preventative measures available.

Essential Fatty Acids (EFAs) could be described as vitamin-like lipids. The body is unable to produce these, yet they are essential for the circulation, body temperature, nerves and protection of tissues, vital for the metabolism and also help our energy level. Essential fatty acids are needed for cell membranes in all the tissues and they also provide a highly reactive action to a group of molecules called the prostaglandins and the leukotrienes. A deficiency of EFAs will soon display itself in a lassitude and a reduced natural immunity, while on the other hand the patient who displayed a good recovery despite having undergone several surgical operations did not have an EFA deficiency because she had regularly used oil of evening primrose capsules.

Deficiencies will affect normal growth; the hair and often the nails will be less healthy; the liver and kidneys will be less effective; the pancreas might suffer and also our energy level will go down and the immune system will suffer. Usually when there is a lack of GLA the skin will become dry and scaly. Now you may well be wondering what relevance this has to the heart or the blood circulation.

I have been outspoken on the fact that I consider that most of the blame for problems in these areas must be apportioned to an imbalance in the diet. Such an imbalance doubtlessly causes deficiencies of vitamins, minerals and/or trace elements, which in turn make our blood circulation less effective. Heart attacks are caused by insufficient blood reaching the heart resulting in an irregular heartbeat. An ineffective blood circulation could well be due to a build-up in a coronary artery resulting in a blocked or restricted blood flow and deposits of fats and cholesterol that then become contributory factors.

We have also read that blood is a slippery liquid and that "PG12" prevents the platelets from sticking to each other or to the artery walls. However, the arteries damaged by deposits of excess fats or cholesterol, high blood pressure or injury, cannot make adequate amounts of PG12. Platelet adhesion to cholesterol deposits rapidly results in blood clots and the flow can easily become blocked or restricted if there is not enough PGE1 and PGE3. The important properties of the GLA contained in oil of evening primrose and in some other seed oils keep the blood slippery and prevent clotting.

It has been said that it was not until 1920 that heart attacks became more prevalent and this has been explained by the changes in our diet. A lack of EFAs resulting from our increasing reliance on processed foods results in vitamin B_6 and vitamin E deficiencies.

As the arteries have a built-in defence system to help themselves, artery spasms will occur more quickly if there are dietary imbalances or deficiencies. The heart is often stronger than we give it credit for, and the heart tissue will not die if there is a temporary blood shortage. However, if the spasms last too long and blood clots do form, then of course the tissue will die. With angina pectoris, for example, where there are partially blocked arteries, emotional stress will place a greater demand on the available oxygen. In these circumstances the patient would be well advised to rest, so that the heart can meet the oxygen requirement. Dilation of the coronary arteries increases the blood flow to help the pain. We see the same effect when patients have to take nitroglycerin, a little tablet that is placed under the tongue, and also PGE1. Many patients have found when they take gamma linoleic acid (GLA) that the severity of an angina attack decreases and that it also reduces the need for the nitroglycerin.

One of the finest remedies is a formula that I have composed myself for such patients. This remedy comprises natural nutrients in a capsulated form; it is called IM nr. and is available in the Nature's Gift range. IM nr. 6 contains high levels of GLA, as among its components it counts the evening primrose seeds, blackcurrant seeds and the scotiaberry, together with some royal jelly and vitamin E. This remedy has proved to be a blessing for many of my patients, not only as a preventative boost to the immune system, but also because it often enables people to reduce their normal drug intake. I have also found IM nr. 6 to be an excellent preventative remedy for heart complaints. The high content of GLA in some of the seeds mentioned above, together with the extra vitamin E, helps the formation of prostacyclin PGL2. This lowers the blood platelet adhesion and increases the effectiveness of cholesterol transportation.

The other combination formula I have introduced into the Nature's Gift range is an oil of evening primrose capsule, combining oil of evening primrose with vitamin C, halibut liver oil, ginseng and zinc. This particular combination, called ADD nr. 4, has brought about great improvements in patients with circulatory problems.

You may well ask why I decided to use fish oils. In recent years scientists have discovered that essential fatty acids (EFAs) are the simplest compounds that can be used for manufacturing other compounds in the body. It is essential that EFAs are included in the diet because they cannot be manufactured in the body. Their importance lies in the fact that they make other necessary compounds, such as prostaglandins and thromboxanes. On the other hand, EFAs are useless unless they can be converted to these other compounds.

While it is true that all EFAs are polyunsaturated, only a few polyunsaturated fatty acids are essential to the diet. In fact, scientists now consider that only linoleic acid is a dietary essential. The body can make certain other vital fatty acids as needed, provided that it is well nourished with vitamins and minerals.

The EFAs are similar to a vitamin. Their absence causes deficiency diseases, just as a vitamin deficiency would. Before the EFAs were isolated and identified, they were actually thought to be vitamins. The designation "vitamin F" was used during the early research, although this term is now obsolete.

I have specifically designed the remedy ADD nr. 4 to improve and increase the rate of distribution and absorption of oil of evening primrose. It is known that GLA and APA (alpha linoleic acid) give better results when combined. This theory was successfully put to the test with harmless experiments on animals, from which it was proved that high blood pressure was quickly regulated. The same outcome is achieved with humans. ADD nr. 4 has also proved its worth when there has been a vascular obstruction.

We have reason to be grateful that in Scotland, in the heart of the Hebrides, a high quality of evening primrose can be found and also some of the berries containing high levels of GLA. I have seen how the great majority of patients who have used the ADD nr. 4 remedy have thrived on the powerful health benefits of these little seeds. Extensive studies have been conducted in this field and on how polyunsaturated fatty acids affect mankind. Every single study has supplied us with more useful knowledge for the prevention of degenerative diseases.

It does not surprise me, when I consider the average standard of dietary management, that deficiencies occur. In today's lifestyle the two types of EFA, namely the Omega 3 series (found in fish oils) and the Omega 6 series (from vegetable origin), have suffered badly. In Eskimo communities the diet still consists predominantly of fish, and there is a very low incidence of heart disease. This again goes to show how relevant our food intake is to our health and how true it is that "we are what we eat".

In the seeds of the evening primrose, this attractive flower, we find a natural substance that cannot be synthesised by the body, but which we can assimilate through a carefully balanced diet. The main dietary EFA, linoleic acid, has to be converted to gamma linoleic acid to be put to full use by the body and therefore together with a good wholesome diet oil of evening primrose will probably help to provide a solution to many of our health problems.

Enough said on the subject of my favourite flower, the evening primrose. There are, of course, other ways also to prevent some of the heart and blood circulatory problems we encounter. Let us turn now to another subject not yet mentioned in any of the previous chapters and that is the fact that trouble with the heart and circulation can be caused by dislocations in the neck, back, spine and/or arms. The blood circulation can be affected by a dislocation and if the body is out of alignment, sometimes a rapid pulse or a missed heartbeat can effectively reduce the usefulness of the red blood corpuscles. It is important for patients with such problems to consult a qualified practitioner. During my career I have dealt with many patients who needed careful adjustment to the neck, spine or back and as a result of manipulation their blood circulation has significantly improved.

Every disc in the body has a specific function and a malfunction of a disc in the cervical or thoracic spine can cause undue pressure on the heart. I have often noticed how much relief heart patients have obtained when this disalignment was carefully adjusted. Moving further down the spine, the lungs can function better after manipulation to rectify a disalignment and a dislocation of the discs of the sacrum could well affect the functioning of the kidneys. Osteopathy or manual therapy can restore the circulation in all these areas, and as the blood is considered the "motor power of the body", it deserves all the encouragement we can give it.

The red corpuscles should be treated as if they were a group of people. They inhabit the arteries and all parts of the circulatory system where the blood flows. In their multiplication they have their own strength and vitality, which they receive from the different hormones in the body. The more work these corpuscles have to do, the faster they will grow until they have matured in size. Then they divide or break away and one part impregnates the other, giving new life to each part and become two red blood corpuscles instead of one. Each corpuscle then goes its own way until it is fully developed, at which time it can again go through the process of division. The blood circulation therefore needs to work in full flow. The food we eat stimulates the blood to a certain extent and when the nutrients are combined with the red and white cells and tissue, the tissue becomes stronger, increasing our vitality.

Our blood count should never be allowed to become low or irregular. If the spine, the hips, the lower limbs and the neck are all working properly and freely, without tension and aches or pains, the circulation will be able to flow more freely thereby alleviating any pressure on the heart. When the circulation is normal the heart will carry out its duties so quietly and smoothly that we will not give it another thought. The condition of the blood influences our disposition, which changes as our blood changes. In my book *Neck and Back Complaints* I have outlined some of the many ways to ensure that our spine is treated with the responsibility and respect it deserves and have suggested several simple methods we can apply to ourselves to improve any problems in this area.

Sometimes it is a good idea to satisfy ourselves that the spine is in the correct position and possibly this relates more to the lumbar spine than any other section. If you discover that one leg is longer than the other you can be sure that there will be a greater degree of involuntary pressure on the arteries, in which case further investigation and treatment will be required. Help can easily be obtained from a qualified practitioner, who will endeavour to rectify the matter and so ensure that you feel better.

Exercise also has a place in a preventative regime; in fact it is essential to maintain good health. If done correctly on a regular basis, exercise will stimulate the metabolism. Physical exercise such as swimming and walking, and even breathing exercises, galvanise the flow of oxygen in the muscular system. Be aware, however, of exercising excessively as this can lead to different problems. Sustained regular and comfortable exercise will invigorate the body.

On the topic of exercise in relation to prevention, I would ask you to answer the following questions:

1. Are you aware of a numbness in your limbs?
2. Do you find that your arms or legs often go to sleep or that you experience "pins and needles"?
3. Do you suffer from cold hands or feet?
4. Do you get cramp in your hand when you write?
5. Do you smoke?
6. Do you drink?
7. Does your job or domestic life cause any stress?
8. Does a short walk cause any aches or pain?
9. Do you drink a lot of coffee or tea, or use other stimulant drinks?

If your answers to the majority of these questions is affirmative, you would be wise to do something about it. Make sure that these apparently minor nuisances do not grow into real problems.

Especially in this day and age, prevention can include the use of supplementary vitamins, minerals and trace elements. An excellent remedy is the Co-Enzyme Q10. I have been most impressed by the work of my dear friend

Dr Len Mervyn, who has done such a marvellous job and really made a breakthrough with the introduction of this excellent formula.

Another excellent preventative remedy is Health Insurance Plus, which is an effective and popular multi-vitamin, mineral and amino acid supplement. It combines thirty-four nutrients in a convenient single tablet and has become a favourite choice of health practitioners, who appreciate the reliability of an all-round supplement that will not interfere with their patients' efforts to maintain good health.

Many supplements cannot be used by people whose vitality is low and who may be sensitive to certain ingredients that are used as the base for concentrated nutrients. In consultation with expert practitioners and in line with the latest research into allergies and sensitivities, Nature's Best has developed a "hypo-allergenic" base for Health Insurance Plus, using only those ingredients that even allergics are least likely to react to. It is guaranteed as being free from wheat, grains, soya, corn, yeast (important especially for people being treated for *Candida albicans*), dairy products and salicylates. It almost goes without saying that sugar and artificial colours, preservatives and flavourings are also excluded. This effort makes Health Insurance Plus ideal for anyone planning to protect their nutritional status by taking a "multi" supplement regularly over a long period of time.

Ultra-trace elements can also serve us well in the case of deficiencies. You may wonder what ultra-trace elements are — the easiest explanation is that they are similar to vitamins. It is only recently that research scientists have discovered how important these tiny mineral elements are for the human system. They now believe that a deficiency of ultra-trace elements may be a contributory cause of certain diseases, especially arteriosclerosis, heart disease and circulatory problems.

In the olden days, when the earth was in ecological balance, there were enough ultra-trace elements in Nature and therefore also in our food. This is now no longer the case. No one in the industrialised countries is receiving sufficient ultra-trace elements. Whether it is summer or winter, whether you are young or old, whether you eat a plain, mixed diet or a vegetarian diet, *everyone* needs a supplement of ultra-trace elements. What are they precisely and why are there not enough in our food today?

The human system has need of both minerals and other inorganic substances, which are received mainly from food, that is from plants and other foodstuffs. Mankind cannot live without the correct nourishment which contains all these inorganic substances. The following elements may be mentioned: carbon, oxygen, nitrogen, phosphorus, potassium, sodium, magnesium and calcium. These are required in large amounts, that is measured in terms of grams or milligrams.

Other basic substances are required only in fractions of a milligram, or microgram doses. (A microgram is one millionth of a gram, that is 0.000001 gram.) On account of the small quantities, and because a few years ago it was impossible to measure them, only small "traces" of these substances could be demonstrated — they were called *trace elements*. The following are some of these trace elements: copper, cobalt, chromium, manganese, molybdenum, nickel, selenium, silicon and zinc.

However, within the last few years, inorganic nutrients have been found in even smaller quantities, and these have therefore been called *ultra-trace* elements. These are in such small quantities that they are measured chiefly in nanograms. (A nanogram is one thousandth of a microgram, that is 0.000.000.001 gram.) Some of these ultra-trace elements are boron, bromide, lithium, rubidium, germanium, arsenic, vanadium, and what are called lanthanides (cerium, dyprosium, erbium, europium, gaolium, holmium, lutetium, neodymium, praseodymium, promethium, samarium, terbium and thulium).

The technology to measure and extract these minute traces has only recently been developed and is a unique and patented process. Research into the importance of ultra-trace elements is still continuing. It is a long, slow process and requires painstaking analysis. However, already four of these ultra-trace elements have been acknowledged as vital, that is essential to good health and found in fairly consistent levels of concentration in all healthy tissue. These four are: boron, bromine, arsenic and vanadium.

It is my professional opinion that many more of the ultra-trace elements will, in time, be widely acknowledged as essential. Among the first to be so recognised will be rubidium, lithium, germanium and the aforementioned lanthanides.

The quantities of trace elements in our diet and their relative proportions are not unimportant. For example, an excess of calcium gives rise to a lack of zinc; too much molybdenum also causes an excess of copper; if one gets too much manganese, a deficiency of magnesium arises. If, for example, one gets too much selenium or cadmium, not to mention arsenic, they will poison the body. What the Swiss physician and alchemist Paracelsus (1493–1541) said applies to these trace elements: "The dose alone decides whether something is poisonous or not."

In order to make the best use of trace elements, it is important that:

1. all the trace elements and ultra-trace elements are present in the diet or dietary supplement;
2. they are present in the correct quantities;
3. they are present in the correct proportions relative to one another;

4. they can be easily absorbed into the human system.

Moreover, for optimal absorption into the system it is necessary for the trace elements to be "amino acid chelated", that is "packed" into amino acids, as is the case in nutritious food.

There are not enough inorganic trace elements and ultra-trace elements in the nourishment that is derived from plants. This is due, in part, to the recent industrialisation of agriculture and horticulture. Methods are being used which bring about a constant reduction of these vital elements. By using ever more concentrated artificial fertilisers, constantly larger crops are being produced, containing smaller and smaller quantities of trace elements. The arable land also becomes exhausted because farmers and market gardeners do not practise the rotation of crops to the same extent as they did formerly.

On account of the lack of trace elements in the soil, the plants become diseased. For example, they lose their ability to protect themselves to the necessary extent against certain parasites. In order to hold their own against these parasites, farmers and market gardeners have to spray their crops with several toxic chemicals, which have negative effects on the plants, the crops and the environment.

Formerly both humans and animals could secure a sufficient supply of minerals, trace elements and ultra-trace elements by eating a balanced, vegetable diet. They can no longer do this.

If the first link in the food chain — plant food — does not contain sufficient trace elements, the next link in the chain — livestock — will also suffer from deficiencies of minerals and trace elements. As a great deal of the common diet depends upon animal products, this deficiency is passed on to humans, along with the damaging effect of the hormones that are used to maximise profits from livestock. Vegetarians also receive too little in the way of trace elements and ultra-trace elements, on account of the shortage in the plant food. In addition, many people nowadays, on account of their sedentary occupation or because of unemployment, do not take in as much nourishment as they did formerly, with the result that they receive even smaller quantities of essential trace and ultra-trace elements.

In many countries, including the United Kingdom, the farming community is firmly convinced of the need to supplement the diet of their livestock with trace elements and ultra-trace elements. The evidence of a deficiency in these essential substances is seen in the common occurrence of various diseases and a higher death rate among livestock. For example, on some farms the death rate among calves and young pigs could be as much as 15 per cent. In some places in the United States, where the soil has been even more systematically exhausted than in most countries, the death rate can be as high as 30 per cent. Mating and gestation problems, anaemia, cardiac degeneration and the so-called "white muscular disease" have been observed among pigs, for example.

What results have livestock breeders achieved by giving their herds supplements of ultra-trace elements? The death rate among livestock has in many cases been reduced from perhaps 15 per cent to 1 per cent, or even less. The sickness rate has likewise been drastically reduced. Mating and gestation problems have been eliminated or most definitely minimised. It is no longer necessary to vaccinate newly born piglets, as they are effectively "vaccinated" through the sows' milk, which contains ultra-trace elements. The cows produce more and better milk. For example, children who are otherwise allergic to milk can readily tolerate milk from cows that receive a supplement of ultra-trace elements. The so-called "white muscular disease" is practically unknown in farms where the feed is enriched with ultra-trace elements, and, on average, the animals to be slaughtered weigh 15 per cent more than animals that have not received a supplement in their feed.

The farmers are glad to have healthy animals — and they also are pleased with the higher profit margins which result. The consumers are also glad to have healthier and better meat and to receive more ultra-trace elements. While many of us may disagree, on both health and ethical grounds, with the large-scale dependence on meat in the diet, it is nevertheless an established part of life for many. It is obvious, even without detailed medical knowledge, that in our modern world we need to supplement our diet with these vital substances from Nature if we are to enjoy good health and maintain a resistance to disease. It is therefore considered advantageous to ensure that we are including in our diet all the trace elements and ultra-trace elements our body needs by taking food supplements which contain all these substances — especially ultra-trace elements — in the correct quantities, in the correct relative proportions and in a formula that can be easily absorbed.

These ultra-trace tablets are imported from Denmark and marketed in this country by Nature's Best, with great results. Again, one cannot go wrong by using these from time to time to ensure the prevention of the problems discussed in this book.

Finally, modern medicine is based on Louis Pasteur's modern theory of disease: "A specific organism causes a specific disease and a specific vaccine gives specific protection." Some shade of doubt exists about this dogma. It has become obvious that for various reasons some individuals have become more susceptible to disease and that the germs themselves simply take advantage of this sensitivity. Some doubts originated when a number of Aboriginal children who had been vaccinated died after the vaccine had been administered. In most cases Pasteur's theory is correct, but in others it clearly is not. One still requires the help of Nature, especially when it comes to prevention.

How invaluable natural remedies are was borne out by a patient who was seriously affected by Raynaud's disease. Amputation was considered essential and this, indeed, appeared to be the logical conclusion. This patient's gangrenous condition was, however, overcome before the surgery took place. A combination of acupuncture, hydrotherapy, vibration and some natural injections was administered and, in this classical case of Raynaud's disease, where circulatory failure was severe, the function was improved to such a degree that amputation could be avoided. This just goes to show how beneficial it can be to give Nature a chance before deciding to finally resort to a more aggressive approach. Surgery should always only be considered as a last resort.

Consider the words of the great scientist Thomas A. Edison, who said that "the doctor of the future will give no medicine, but will interest his patients in the care of the human frame, in diet and in the cause and prevention of disease".

12

Helpful Hints

IS THE DIET really so all-important for circulatory problems? I would say that it is indeed one of the most important factors as this is where it all begins. If the daily diet is modified, the patient will immediately notice a change in his or her condition. The more healthy the diet, the more essential nutrients it will contain. Long-standing deficiencies need immediate attention and action. Make a habit of reading the labels of the items you select from the shelves in the supermarket.

Toxicity of the blood will impede the circulation and in such cases a detoxification programme will be useful. I have already mentioned some suitable programmes along with an outline for fasting, which gives a similar result. However, even if wholesome food is available, the method of preparation is also important. Aluminium pots and pans, pressure cookers and microwave ovens should be avoided. Also be wary of artificial additives.

An excellent book for general dietary guidelines is *The Liver, the Regulator of Your Health* by Dr A. Vogel, and one that is more specifically related to the subject in hand is *Don't Eat Your Heart Out* by Joseph C. Piscatella. You will find a great amount of helpful nutritional advice in these books, and the general diet outlined in Chapter 3 will also serve you well.

I have already mentioned the little-known properties of oats and the following recipe for preparing oats has been handed down for generations and adapted so that as little nutritional value is lost in the preparation as possible.

> 2 fl oz cut oats
> 2 fl oz Miller's pure oat bran
> 1 fl oz unsalted raisins (no preservatives)
> 1 fl oz unsalted currants (no preservatives)
> 8 fl oz of spring water

Preheat a thermos flask by filling with boiling water and sealing. Add the raisins and currants to the spring water in a stainless steel pan and heat to boiling point. Mix the oats and oat bran (dry), empty the thermos flask then place the dry mix inside, quickly add the boiling water with the raisins and currants and seal. The mixture may be eaten with a long-handled spoon directly from the thermos flask any time from thirty minutes to four hours later. Thoroughly rinse the thermos flask with cold water to clean. This mixture can be made first thing in the morning and eaten when desired. The oatmeal can also be prepared in the usual way using a pot on the cooker, or if need be in a pressure cooker, but the method described above is preferable.

Oat bran is valuable for any of the complaints dealt with in this book. To reap the maximum benefits from this, it is necessary to consume roughly 2–3 ounces of oat bran a day. It can also be sprinkled over meals or snacks, but always make sure that you use good quality oats. The difference between oat bran and other types of bran is that oat bran contains a large proportion of soluble fibre, whereas other types contain more insoluble fibres. Of course, it does no good to go overboard, and think that this will be the complete answer to the problem. It is often advisable to take along with the oat bran some vitamin B_3 (niacin), especially in the case of a high cholesterol count.

I would like to stress once more that junk food and packaged food should always be avoided. Common sense will tell you what is best for you and nearly always that will be freshly prepared and natural food without any chemical additives.

Adopt a positive mental attitude. For the physical aspect think about exercise, recreation, meditation or manipulation. Nutritionally, pay attention to diet, vitamins, minerals, trace elements and herbs. This is the best advice anyone can give you.

The real threats for the problems discussed in this book are sugar, salt, animal fats, starches, nicotine and alcohol and these ought to be avoided where possible. If you just think that since the early nineteenth century the average person's consumption of sugar has increased from 10 lbs per year to 140 lbs per year, you will realise what we are asking our bodies to cope with.

It is also good to try and bring some variety into the diet. Ensuring that the amount of cholesterol is kept as low as possible does not mean that the diet has to be boring; there are plenty of other foods available from which to choose attractive meals.

Relatively minor dietary adjustments may help to reduce the astronomically high figure of 50,000 people dying prematurely of heart disease in the United Kingdom every year. Professor David Galton and his team from St Bartholomew's Hospital in London has said that although smoking, high blood cholesterol and being overweight do increase the risk of having a heart attack, one of the most important predictors is having a first-degree relative who has suffered a heart attack before the age of fifty-five. Through practical screening programmes it will be possible to identify those people who are most at risk and help them with vigorous and appropriate treatment. This information comes from the Nutritional Information Service, and again shows how much diet is involved.

Please make sure that you eat sufficient fresh foods, salads and vegetables and that there is enough fibre in your food. Preferably use bottled water, bran, oats, nuts, honey, cottage cheese and yoghurt and please do not forget unpolished rice.

Instead of vinegar it is advisable to use Molkosan, from Bioforce. Molkosan contains the whey of the milk, is practically free of fat and contains two very important proteins, albumen and globulin, which are the two main constituents of the human blood plasma. Furthermore, Molkosan contains the trace element orotic acid, which has an active influence. Whey is also rich in natural lactose, which is quickly absorbed into the digestive system and helps to maintain a good intestinal flora. Molkosan eliminates excess water, stimulates the liver and helps the inflammatory processes, but its most important effects in the context of the problems under discussion here are that it assists the cellular respiration and through its high mineral content improves the blood circulation. It also reduces the cholesterol content in the blood and therefore has an antisclerotic effect. This product can be used to make a very tasty salad dressing and I must stress how beneficial it can be. The recommended substitute for table salt is Herbamare sea salt.

The following is a checklist of practical advice provided by the International Society of Cardiology:

* Exercises should be done carefully and they are better done before work in the morning than after work at night.
* Walking is a very good exercise and it would pay to make this into a regular habit.

* Maintaining a reasonable level of physical fitness is better than excessive exercising or following a strenuous athletic programme.
* A regular exercising routine is very much more valuable than sudden bursts of strenuous exercise.
* Do not exercise for at least two hours after a big meal.
* Do not exercise if you are feeling unwell or overtired.
* Do not lift weights above your powers — rather, wait until someone else can assist you.
* While on holiday enjoy some gentle extra exercise, such as swimming.
* If you experience angina problems, breathlessness or palpitations, stop and rest and always take care not to overdo exercises.
* Have a good rest after your exercise.
* If you want to take a bath after you have exercised make sure that the water is nice and warm.
* Should you experience any lightheadedness, palpitations, giddiness or heaviness in the legs, please consult your doctor.
* If you experience any pain in the joints because of excessive work or exercising, allow yourself a rest and reduce the intensity of the exercise programme.
* Have a regular check-up with your doctor or practitioner, who will advise you further.

It will also be beneficial to take some homoeopathic or natural remedies for your specific complaints. Carry them with you and if you are already on drugs, with the help of your doctor you may just be able to reduce some of your drug intake in order to let the body take over again.

Acupuncture, osteopathy or naturopathy may also give your body the help it needs to perform correctly.

One of the most important factors nowadays, especially for the heart patient, is this fashionable word "stress". The stress factor in today's society can often present a serious health threat. To relieve stress or anxieties, scrutinise your lifestyle. Many people are no longer able to recognise stress as it has become part of their life. If stress is leading to fear, unpleasant emotions or worry, then some action must be taken to relieve or control it and in so doing help the anxiety and tension which prevents the body from doing its job to its best ability.

A serious look at oneself is necessary, and always remember that help is available from natural remedies, herbal remedies or flower remedies.

Allow yourself a little time to listen to your body and during mealtimes train yourself to take the time to chew the food properly, because by overloading ourselves with too much food, we will ultimately be heading for disaster.

Wherever possible, avoid spending long periods under artificial lights or in excessively noisy surroundings and, especially, give your car a rest now and then. Do not forget that oxygen is a vital necessity and especially during breathing exercises make sure that you inhale deeply through the nose. Stretch, loosen yourself, exhale and inhale deeply and, whatever exercise you take, try if at all possible to perform it in the fresh air and the body will feel revitalised.

An evaluation of one's lifestyle followed by the necessary adjustments could well be more effective than any other approach to treatment. It is a well-known fact that heart patients in particular can become quite emotional and easily upset. This can be greatly helped with herbal remedies such as *Avena sativa*, an oat extract from the Bioforce range, as this will help to alleviate the underlying tension. Patients with heart disorders are also likely to worry more. Thoughts like "When will my heart stop beating?" and "How long do I still have to live?" will always lurk in the back of the mind. This tendency is something that should be overcome because it will nearly always make the condition worse and definitely not better. We are full of fears: the fear of not being correct, the fear of being that little bit different, the fear of becoming poor, the fear of not being accepted. Let us try to be natural and take an interest in what happens around us — an interest in the frightening as well as the interesting and fascinating things in the world. Do not dwell too much on what other people think of you, because it does not really matter. Learn to live with yourself and enjoy life. The quality of life will be expressed in our state of health.

Worry is one of the worst toxins there is. The greatest worry is fear and nothing lowers our vitality more than becoming fearful. It is no good thinking that we have a problem and we had better learn to live with it. That problem should not change our way of thinking, but should change our actions.

A more successful approach is not to sit back and wallow in our problems, but to think of how we can start to do something about them. Wishful thinking will not achieve anything. The harassed lives that many of us lead in order to meet our own and someone else's expectations make it essential that we try to achieve harmony in mind and body. Again I wish to stress that it is better not to dwell on the past; instead, look forward positively to the future and appreciate what it may have to offer. Positive thoughts can only enhance the situation. Remember what our mothers and grand-mothers taught us when we were young: it is good to occasionally stop and listen to the voice in our heart and this instinct will steer us in the right direction to correct the disharmony which today's lifestyle is trying to take away from us. I hope that this book may be of help in relieving some of the suffering and improve the quality of your life and your health.

Bibliography

Dr Morton Walker, *Chelation Therapy,* Freelance Communications, Connecticut, USA.

Irene Stein, *Royal Jelly,* Thorsons Publishing Group, Wellingborough, Northants.

Roger Newman Turner, ND, DO, BAc, *Angina,* Thorsons Publishing Group, Wellingborough, Northants.

Judy Graham, *Evening Primrose Oil,* Thorsons Publishing Group, Wellingborough, Northants.

Dr Carolyn Shreeve, *A Healthy Heart for Life,* Thorsons Publishing Group, Wellingborough, Northants.

Bircher Benner, *Hartpatienten,* De Driehoek, Amsterdam, the Netherlands.

Thorwald Dethlefsen Rudiger Dahlke, *De Zin van Ziekzijn,* Uitgevery Ankh Hermes, Deventer, the Netherlands.

Alfred Vogel, *Nature, Your Guide to Healthy Living,* A. Vogel Verlag, Teufen, Switzerland.
The Liver, the Regulator of Your Health, A. Vogel Verlag, Teufen, Switzerland.
The Nature Doctor: A Manual of Traditional Medicine, Mainstream Publishing, Edinburgh.

Dr Ian Anderson, *Heart Attacks Understood,* Pan Books, London.

Dr James J. Julian MD, *Chelation Extends Life,* Welness Press, Holywood, USA.

Joseph C. Piscatella, *Don't Eat Your Heart Out,* Thorsons Publishing Group, Wellingborough, Northants.

Dr Richard A. Passwater, *Evening Primrose Oil — Its Amazing Nutrients and the Health Benefits They Can Give You,* Keats Publishing Inc., Connecticut, USA.